MEDICAL SCHOOL:
GETTING IN,
STAYING IN,
STAYING HUMAN

MEDICAL SCHOOL: GETTING IN, STAYING IN, STAYING HUMAN

Keith R. Ablow

 WILLIAMS & WILKINS
Baltimore • London • Los Angeles • Sydney

Editor: Nancy Collins
Associate Editor: Carol Eckhart
Copy Editor: Marylane Soeffing
Design: Alice Sellers
Production: Anne G. Seitz
Managing Editor: Linda Napora

Copyright © 1987
Williams & Wilkins
428 East Preston Street
Baltimore, MD 21202, U.S.A.

Printed in the United States of America

Library of Congress Cataloging-in-Publication Data

Ablow, Keith R.
  Medical School: Getting In, Staying In, Staying Human.

  1. Medical colleges—Admission.   2. Premedical
education.   I. Title.   [DNLM: 1. Education, Premedical.
2. Educational Measurement.   3. Schools, Medical.
W 18 A152m]
R838.4.A25   1987   610'.7'11   86-15646
ISBN 0-683-00004-7

Printed at the Waverly Press, Inc.

87 88 89 90 91   10 9 8 7 6 5 4 3 2 1

To my mother, father, and sister—
evergreens in the dead of winter.

Foreword

Keith Ablow has the happy ability to be involved in events and, at the same time, be witness to them. As I write this, he is about to begin his fourth year in the School of Medicine of the Johns Hopkins University. I have known him during those first three years and I've had the chance, too, to read all of the information we have accumulated in his file; the application to medical school, the recommendation letters, the interview notes made by the senior physician whom he met during the admissions process. In addition to our many conversations, I have also his writings. I have learned that Keith is quite obviously extraordinarily bright and deeply committed to service. He is sincere, honest and insightful. The readers of this book will suspect that he is also something of a pragmatist, but that his pragmatism and even a faint suspicion of cynicism do not dilute for one moment the idealistic purposes.

In fact, the casual reader of this book might react negatively to the evident "gamesmanship" as Keith leads the tyro through the hedgerows of application to medical school. I would not adopt that point of view; rather, I see what Keith offers as a lesson in the pragmatic pursuit of a worthy goal—and becoming a physician is a worthy goal.

Indeed, the processes we have set up in the colleges and universities of the United States have forced the need for pragmatism. And, while I would not agree with Keith that all of the root of the "pre-med syndrome" derives from those processes, I do agree that the young student desiring to become a physician must understand the demands of the pathway if there is to be success. I don't have the space in which to dissect this argument thoroughly but I would remind of just one fact. Each medical school has an application fee. The cost of application alone for most students can add up to hundreds of dollars. There are practical issues.

Much more importantly, Keith has not ignored the broad range of concern. His title—*Medical School: Getting In, Staying In, Staying Human*—reminds us of that. There is a wealth of insight and a great deal of practical advice. There is also quite evident attention to and suggestion about approaches to the preservation of perspective and of calm and equanimity during an often trying process. Keith has recognized this need and he serves it well. He has provided a guide and not a straitjacket, and he always allows plenty of room for the "self" of the applicant to be preserved.

In sum, then, it is a privilege to have had the opportunity to write this brief introduction and to commend this book to those who have the worthy goal of becoming a physician.

Henry M. Seidel, M.D.
Associate Dean for Student Affairs
The Johns Hopkins University
School of Medicine

Preface

*"The credit belongs to the man who is actually in the arena
... who knows the great enthusiasm, the great devotions, and
spends himself in a worthy cause."*

THEODORE ROOSEVELT

Your acceptance to medical school will be the result of years of hard work. You will, perhaps, have put in far more study time than many of your friends. You will have completed a myriad of required premedical courses, suffered through the Medical College Admission Test (MCAT), and wrestled with the medical school application process itself. The price tag—in time, discipline, and dollars—will have been staggering.

I made that investment, too. I'm sure I spent more time in Brown University's Rockefeller Library than I did in my dorm room. I cancelled my share of dates before organic chemistry and physics exams. And it paid off when The Johns Hopkins School of Medicine admitted me to the class of 1987.

One of the reasons that all the preparation and sacrifice proved worthwhile is that I took advantage of advice from deans, physicians, and medical students who knew some of the intricacies of the medical school admissions process. I didn't make the mistakes they warned against, and, with this book, neither will you. If you have the necessary dedication to achieve the goal of attending medical school, the following pages will help you clear many of the hurdles.

This is not a cookbook. I refused one friend's good-natured advice that I write "something really basic with lots of lists." There are enough address books masquerading as helpful guides without adding another to the pile. That's why this book begins with a consideration of whether medical school and medicine (the two are not at all alike) are really for you. If I've succeeded, you'll put this book down at least a few times as you flip from page to page. You'll want to think whether it's all really worth it to you. You may even get a little confused. Good. The only way to become a good doctor, and to convince admissions committees that you'd make one, is to have wrestled with your motivations. In many ways, confronting your own doubts is like running—it may hurt while you're doing it, but it feels great when you break the tape at the finish line.

The following chapters will help you to make decisions and will give you specific guidelines to follow at the high school, college, and, since I share your hopes for success, medical school levels. They will give you a head start toward choosing an undergraduate school, structuring your premedical curriculum, preparing for the MCAT, writing your medical school applications, interviewing, and making it through the four tough years that will follow your acceptance.

Medical School: Getting In, Staying In, Staying Human has another agenda. I am close enough to my years of premedical and medical education to understand just how stressful they can be. Dealing with that stress and completing the educational process with your sensitivity and outside interests intact—as a whole person—is more important than your test scores in biology and anatomy. I have been careful to address the strengths and weaknesses of premedical and medical education and to offer advice that I hope will help you deal with the shortcomings of each.

I believe that you will keep this book for many years. I would also like to think that copies will find their way into the hands of medical students who would profit from much of what I have to say. High school guidance counselors, premedical advisors, undergraduate professors, and medical school educators and administrators would also benefit from reading through all 10 chapters. The medical school admissions process should be the result of an integration of perspectives at many levels of the ordeal.

Finally, I want to wish you luck. I remember my own anxieties at each of the steps that I'm going to help you through. I must have gone to my mailbox five times a day before an acceptance letter from Hopkins arrived. It wasn't easy, and many times it wasn't fun, but the admissions game can be won, and you've already got the playbook in hand.

Acknowledgments

I would like to acknowledge the interest of Howard Baum, Abraham Kader, and Douglas Lakin who took the time to read and comment on parts of this book and whose friendship will be my most treasured memory of medical school.

Medical School: Getting In, Staying In, Staying Human has also benefited from the valued input of the editors of Williams & Wilkins. Nancy McSherry-Collins, Linda Napora, Carol Eckhart, Anne Seitz, and John Gardner each have my sincere appreciation.

My thanks to Dr. Henry Seidel, Associate Dean for Student Affairs at The Johns Hopkins University School of Medicine, not only for providing the foreword to this book, but also for his guidance, his friendship, and the example of his character.

My thanks also to Dr. Norman Anderson, Assistant Dean for Admission, for reviewing and commenting on each chapter. He and his staff were instrumental in providing the sample essays included in Chapter 6.

Finally, I thank Dr. Peter Dans, Dr. Stuart Fine, Dr. Lawrence Grouse, and Dr. Arthur Ulene for their warm support and valued advice over the past four years.

Contents

1

Deciding to Be a Physician

*"In the practical decisions of life it will scarcely ever be
possible to go through all the arguments in favor of or
against one possible decision, and one will, therefore, always
have to act on insufficient evidence. . . . Even the most
important decisions in life must always contain this inevitable
element of irrationality"* (1).

WERNER HEISENBERG

ALL ABOUT PATIENCE

One of the most valuable skills an individual can possess, and which, unfortunately, usually comes later in life, is patience. Patience, to my mind, means being honest enough with yourself to put off important decisions until you have gathered sufficient information to make them wisely.

The temptation to choose medicine as a career early on—perhaps during your sophomore or junior year in high school—comes from all the transient rewards you would receive by committing to a field so quickly. You could start enjoying the praise of your parents and their friends right away. You could avoid all those career counseling workshops at your high school or college. And, you wouldn't be subject to the frowns you might well have received from your teachers if you had told them that you didn't know what you wanted to become.

But, be careful. Such rewards don't last very long. They're hardly worth agonizing through premedical courses you really have no interest in. And they're certainly no bargain if they're followed by a career you hate waking up to every morning. It's important to be honest with yourself at every step of the process of becoming a physician. If you have doubts, rest assured that they are normal. Whether in high school, college, or medical school there are ways, discussed throughout this book, to gather any additional information you need to make a well-grounded judgment about where you should be headed.

Until you have all the information you need to feel comfortable, you may find it easier to tell others that you "have an interest in medicine." Explain to them that you want to make very sure that your profession will be enjoyable and fulfilling for you. The people who truly care about you won't flash any frowns. And, even if they do let slip an occasional disappointed sigh, remember that you alone will have to pay the price for hasty commitments. Keep your eyes open. Explore.

KEEPING PARENTAL AND PEER
INFLUENCE IN PERSPECTIVE

My parents are very honest people. So honest, in fact, that I can often read their happiness, disappointment, or anger just by a determined glance past their glasses. So they didn't have to say anything at all in order for me to tell they were disappointed when, during my junior year at Brown, I questioned my earlier decision to become a physician and began to look into careers other than medicine.

It wasn't that they didn't want me to be happy. It wasn't that I would be abandoning any family tradition in medicine—there is none. What it was was a very understandable reaction to a possible loss. For a few years already, after all, they had expected that their son would become a doctor. He would someday be secure financially, enjoy the respect of the community, perhaps even teach at a university. The thought of losing all that hurt, and it showed in their eyes.

Your parents are probably no different than mine. Many of them may never have had the opportunity to receive a professional education. With the chance they have given you to study medicine, they may think that you are callous or unappreciative if you choose another path. They may even feel that they have failed in attempting to ensure the success of the next generation. If either of your parents is a physician, he or she may see your indecision as a negative judgment on him or herself.

Don't get angry. Try to understand that parents make large investments in their children, but have frustratingly little control on the return once their sons and daughters begin to make independent decisions. Explain that you are not making a choice between being lazy and working hard, but, rather, choosing which field can most completely command your deep devotion. Invite them to explore with you the various careers you might be considering. Don't let them feel that they are losing their investment; make them partners.

In addition to your parents, your friends will almost certainly offer their perspectives on whether you should be a doctor. Keep in mind that your high school or college contemporaries probably have no more information about the medical profession than you do. They are often poor judges of whether your talents and tastes or, for that matter, your grades and scores are well-suited for a particular career. Listen, and thank them for their interest in your future, but don't turn on or turn off to medicine based on their well-intentioned friendly advice.

On the other hand, always be willing to listen. If may indeed be your parents who rightly point out that many of your interests seem to mesh with the medical profession. Or it might be a close friend who first asks you directly whether you're "premed" because you want to be or because your father wants you to be. There are some individuals with special insight into you as a person. They can be valuable resources, but only if you take the additional step of thinking critically about what they have to say.

GATHERING INFORMATION

During the early phase of deciding to be a physician, a realistic goal is to get a flavor of medicine as a career. Understand that a final verdict on your happiness as a healer may not, even with the best-researched decision, come until you are further along in the educational process. You will find increasingly wide windows through which to look into the medical profession as you progress through premedical and medical education. There are, however, keyholes it would be wise to peek through long before you send for your applications.

Private physicians are an invaluable resource. Most, especially those who have gotten to know you as a patient or neighbor, will be willing, even flattered, to discuss the medical profession with you. Call, make an appointment, and ask the tough questions. Ask what a typical day is like, what kinds of hours he or she puts in, whether he feels fulfilled when his head hits the pillow at night, what he might have done differently, what opportunities are still open to him. And don't be afraid to ask if you seem well-suited for medicine. Remember, though, filter what you hear on a very fine screen.

If you feel that physicians you know personally may not be candid with you in their appraisals of the medical profession, call doctors outside of your hometown. You may want to contact the American Medical Association or the public relations office of a nearby hospital. They can often suggest a physician who would be willing to meet with a student considering a career in medicine. Or, if you come across an interesting newspaper or magazine article on medicine written by an MD, you can contact the author. He or she may not have the time to bat all your ideas around with you, but you might come away with some valuable advice.

In addition to talking your thoughts through with medical professionals, you should try to arrange a day or two to "shadow" willing physicians. Doctors work in diverse environments including hospitals, private offices, and research laboratories. Each setting has its own flavor, and you can begin to appreciate the breadth of the profession by spending time in more than one environment. You may even be able to find a single physician who, because he divides his time between patient care and laboratory research, can help you learn about multiple facets of medicine.

One potential obstacle you may encounter, perhaps unknowingly, is what I like to call the "postmed syndrome." Successful physicians are notorious for letting the rigors of medical training slip their minds as more and more years pass. To get an immediate viewpoint on what premedical and medical education is like, contact the Dean of Student Affairs at the medical school nearest your home. Request the names of a few students with whom you could speak. And, again, ask tough questions. Has it been worth it? Would you do it over again? How does family life fit into your plans? What are the qualities you like about your classmates and instructors? What are the qualities you least like?

I don't think that any of the physicians and students I spoke with before medical school offered his or her time hesitantly. Most medical students and doctors will have given much thought to the long road they have traveled and have yet to travel. They enjoy offering an interested individual some of what they have learned. Listen carefully and you may avoid critical mistakes.

After gathering information in these limited ways, you may want to commit more time—a summer or longer—to work in a local hospital or to participate in medical research. The chapters that follow will explain the best ways to set up such a summer experience. Of course, if you follow the suggestions above, you'll already know a few medical professionals who may be willing to help you find a stimulating environment in which to work. Don't be shy.

WHAT TO EXPECT OF THE EDUCATIONAL PROCESS

One of the most important understandings to which you will come is that premedical education and the first two years of medical education bear little or no resemblance to the practice of medicine. This makes the insight you gain from physicians and medical students even more important. They can help to provide the motivation necessary for you to excel academically now or in coming years. There are things about the educational process itself, however, that may bear on your decision to pursue a medical career.

The requirements for entry to medical school generally include one year of introductory biology, one year of physics, and one year each of inorganic and organic chemistry. Many schools require, or strongly suggest, additional courses in English and math. While the specifics of structuring a successful premedical program are presented in Chapter 3, you should already realize that "being premed" means not being a lot of other things. With so much science to learn there is less time for deep exploration of the humanities. Science can be dry. Organic chemistry is more factual than it is intellectual, and physics requires abstract mathematical modes of thought which are wholly alien to literary analysis. You may or may not love such courses. You must be able to tolerate them. They have nothing to do with doctoring, but they have everything, under the present system, to do with getting the chance to learn how to doctor. Moreover, if the best you can do is tolerate your premedical coursework, resenting all the while the fact that you are sacrificing other disciplines you love, your college years may well be unhappy ones. Stop to think how much weight you put on final goals relative to your contentment while achieving them. How important is your happiness on the road to a career? Can you achieve the necessary grades in courses you don't enjoy?

The premedical years can be highly pressurized. More students than can be admitted to medical school want to go, and you may be faced with intensely competitive, genuinely serious, young men and women as classmates. You will spend long laboratory sessions with them. You will be in study groups with them. You will be graded on a curve with them. The premedical years are not years through which you can coast. Even the most talented students work hard. If that sounds like a nightmare to you, think of something else to study.

Don't be fooled by the "light at the end of the tunnel" mirage. Many of my friends at Brown thought that the toughest years were over once they were accepted to medical school. Wrong. The preclinical years at many American medical schools are much more demanding than any premedical program. The work is harder, the hours are longer (class may last from 9 a.m. to 5 p.m. every day), and the competition is stiffer. While some medical schools have integrated glimpses of clinical medicine into their first year curriculum, most of the substance of the first year is hard, basic science—biochemistry, anatomy, physiology. If you understand that you won't be touching a stethoscope for quite some time, you may find the process less frustrating.

Very few students enjoy the first year of medical school.

Many of them call it the worst year of their lives. For those who only tolerated premedical science courses, the first year of medical school is a bitter pill. The sociology course they lived for is over. There are no classroom debates about politics or religion. What they find are textbooks and slides and cadavers. In the second year and thereafter, the courses are more relevant. Disease processes are introduced and contact with patients is increased. By the third year, all the students' time is spent working in the hospital setting—assisting in surgery, learning the intricacies of diagnosis, becoming proficient at physical examination. The training for one's life work begins in earnest, and it can be invigorating. But it is not easy. The goal of becoming a competent physician translates to large amounts of time spent assimilating facts and figures about various disease states. There are nights without sleep spent caring for patients.

Following your completion of medical school, most states require that you work as a medical resident in a hospital for two to six years, depending upon the particular area of medicine that you would like to enter. Your income during these years may be only $20,000, and your work week may reach 100 hours. While these years provide experience which serves as the foundation for physicians' careers, most residents find at least some periods of their training extremely stressful. If you harbor doubts about your direction, you must clear them before signing on for such a concentrated and demanding program.

You will have to decide yourself, with the limited amount of information you have, whether the payback will be worth the investment. If you enjoy studying science and if you thrive on competition, your investment will be a more pleasant and less risky one. But if you're bored with science and become unhappy when competition is stiff, stop several times during the years to come and think whether it's all worth it to you. Remember that your assessment will be more difficult since the work required in college and medical school doesn't reflect the reality of medical practice. Your goal in becoming a physician is to help people, not to memorize tables of useless anatomical minutiae.

Hating anatomy, organic chemistry, or even your surgical rotation doesn't mean you won't love being a pediatrician.

INCOME, PROFESSIONAL FLEXIBILITY, AND JOB SATISFACTION OF PHYSICIANS

According to the American Medical Association, the average net income (before taxes) of physicians in the United States was $108,400 in 1984 (2). An average generally means that many individuals fell below, and many stood above, the reported value. There are doctors who earn less than $40,000. Some earn $500,000. Much of the discrepancy arises from choices medical professionals make as various opportunities arise. Those who feel comfortable in an academic environment may be willing to forego a large income in order to teach or do research. Some dedicated individuals may choose to practice in poor or sparsely populated areas. Others may give higher priority to financial success. Such physicians may structure large, lucrative practices, often in specialties such as plastic surgery or ophthalmology, which allow them to earn as much as executives of the largest corporations in America. As things stand today, the money is there if you want it and are willing to work for it.

Along with relative financial security, the physician enjoys great professional flexibility. Graduating MDs may choose from specialty training in systems as diverse as the brain (neurology and neurosurgery), the female reproductive system (obstetrics and gynecology), and the skeleton (orthopedic surgery). There are more than 20 recognized medical specialties, and new areas are developing all the time. The young physician may also opt for a career that includes medical research, hospital administration, or teaching. It is possible to participate in public health work or government programs. Law firms and the finance industry increasingly utilize graduating physicians as advisors on issues involving medicine and the law or medicine and technology.

For professionals who desire a change later in life, many of the same paths remain open. It is possible to receive training in an additional specialty of medicine, to work toward a degree in public health, or to begin teaching. There is no mandatory age for physician retirement. There is often no critical eye watching the quality of the work he performs. The physician may choose to take on young associates to lighten the load as work hours begin to weigh too heavily.

Still, some of the more than 50 physicians with whom I have spoken say that they would choose another career given the chance to do things over again. Many express their dissatisfaction by strongly discouraging their children from entering the medical profession. There are several reasons for the apparent discontent. First, some of those I asked actually made it through the rigors of medical education and residency training even though they disliked the material that they were being taught. For them, the excitement of being at one's life's work never took hold. They ignored their own instincts, and, having invested more and more time to climb each rung of the ladder to a medical career, they lost sight of the ground. To turn back would be a terrible waste, they feared. And, now, with even more years invested, they are unhappy and unfulfilled.

Second, physicians are not a humble lot. A great many people, in a wide variety of professions, never attain the complete success for which they had hoped. Some doctors, however, have the tendency to blame faded dreams on their choice of a career. If they had become businessmen, they theorize, vast financial empires would have come under their control. Such individuals may have done better or worse in another line of work. It's comforting for them to think they would have done better in another profession, but it may not be true.

Third, really content and satisfied people are rare. It may be that doctors are representative of all highly motivated individuals. Perhaps life really does not hold enough for many of us. What is encouraging is that so many of the physicians with whom I spoke did feel fulfilled. They expressed the excitement of continuing intellectual growth and professional advancement. Many felt that curing illness and prolonging human life were the most basic and vital endeavors they could imagine anyone undertaking.

Finally, the most frequent warning issued by the satisfied and discontent alike was that medicine is changing and that those qualities of the profession that they most closely embraced are under siege.

HOW MEDICINE MAY CHANGE

The greatest concern generated by new trends in medicine seems to revolve around the physician's loss of autonomy and independence. Increasingly, our society has decided to place medicine in the marketplace. Large for-profit corporations control more and more of the industry that is medicine. Patients increasingly seek care in free-standing emergency clinics and private hospitals. As Arnold Relman, MD, Editor of *The New England Journal of Medicine* put it, "If we cling to our present course, I am convinced that the independence and ethical base of our profession will be progressively eroded and the practice of medicine will continue to evolve into commerce (3, p 18)." Already, he notes, 50 percent of all physicians are paid on a salary, rather than fee-for-service basis.

Added to this threat to the medical professional's independence is increasing competition between physicians, fueled by a surplus of doctors in the United States. By the year 1990, the Graduate Medical Education National Advisory Committee (GMENAC) estimates that there will be 70,000 more physicians than the country needs. Competition from nurse practitioners, chiropractors, osteopaths, and podiatrists is likely to expand. With more players in the health care game, doctors may find it more difficult to reach the high income brackets.

Competition has already brought advertising and marketing into medicine; these aspects of current practice may be unattractive to you. For example, an article in *Michigan Medicine* advises:

> A listing of all private practitioners, PAs, HMOs, hospital services and free-standing clinics that offer—or may offer—services similar to those provided by the physician's practice is important. Where possible, identify by name the physicians and key paramedical professionals involved in these services. . . . Summarize the strengths and weaknesses of each service and estimate the number of patients that they serve (4).

The costs of marketing and advertising, along with the investment necessary to keep pace with medical technology's newfangled procedures and equipment, will make it more difficult for doctors choosing to practice alone. Large group practices and multispecialty clinics, enjoying the advantages of pooled resources and shared expenses, will also have an impact on the independence of solo practitioners.

Because physicians themselves have been unable to control the costs of health care, government agencies may be forced to regulate more strictly the fees physicians charge and, perhaps, the areas in which they practice. Insurance companies have begun to limit the tests and extended hospital stays doctors may feel are necessary for their patients. Today, there may be a one-time standard reimbursement to the hospital for the patient with a particular diagnosis. Physicians have to be more selective in the procedures they order so as not to exceed the standard amount and, thereby, undermine the cost-effectiveness programs in their hospitals or institutions.

Beyond increasing competition and outside regulation, the medical profession is becoming more highly technical and specialized. Nearly 70 percent of practicing physicians in the

United States decide against general or family practice, becoming instead internists, anesthesiologists, neonatologists, and practitioners of other highly specialized disciplines (3). More and more patients are now cared for by "experts" on a particular anatomical region. If your heart is set on general practice, you may not treat the wide range of interesting disorders that once fell in the domain of general medicine.

What I've said may encourage or discourage you. You may feel that the marketing of medicine has been a long time in coming. It may provide an outlet for your business savvy that you feared would never come into play. Whatever your reaction, bear in mind that the truly dedicated physician can still choose from many paths. The most traditional paths, however, will become even more difficult to travel.

THE RIGHT REASONS AND THE WRONG REASONS

Though I didn't mention it in the preface, this book is also not a code of ethics. The right reasons for becoming a physician include any and every one of your true motivations that can actually be realized through a career in medicine. I will not attempt to judge your particular goals—you must come to terms with what you're after and why.

Affluence and prestige, for example, are certainly among the rewards attainable through a career in medicine. Doctors are among the highest paid individuals in the United States, and they make their money, for the most part, by helping others. In doing so, they often win the respect of the community. The fact that an MD has completed a program of education widely known to be rigorous adds to the admiration many feel for physicians.

Medicine is also an unusually safe profession to enter. Unlike recently graduated lawyers or business professionals, young doctors are still assured of relatively high incomes should they desire such financial rewards and remain dedicated to their work. The risks inherent in accepting a position in the lowest echelon of a law firm or in starting a business are much greater. Those who finish at the bottom of their law school class, in fact, may find themselves unemployed following graduation.

The problem with using money, status, and security as goals is that they tend to be relatively weak motivators. The process of becoming a physician is so expensive, so consuming, and so difficult that, with no higher ideals for which to strive, you will almost certainly give up the fight during either your premedical, medical school, or, worse yet, your residency years. Moreover, if you have the intelligence to make it far along the road to a career in medicine, chances are you could have beaten the odds in business or another field and climbed high on the financial totem pole. Becoming a plastic surgeon may take ten years following college graduation. That's ten years you could have used to inch up the corporate ladder.

Stronger motivations tend to include a large measure of the basic desire to serve. Many of my classmates are motivational hybrids of a sort. They enjoy nice clothing, they want to travel, and they hope to be able to offer their children the best education their intelligence and determination allow. But they also feel a strong need to help others. Alleviating suffering appeals to them on a basic, human level. It's what they believe will allow them to sleep contentedly at night and to look back when they are sixty or seventy years old and feel that life has been worthwhile. It's also the only thing that really carries them through the sleepless nights working on hospital wards.

Some students also see medicine as satisfying their intense intellectual curiosity. Personal interaction with patients is sometimes less important to them. They embrace medical science and enjoy the constant challenge of pushing back the boundaries of medical knowledge. They may, in fact, find the process of becoming a physician invigorating rather than taxing. They love to learn.

Again, be honest with yourself. As I have already discussed, the only motivations that will surely lead to unhappiness are those that you allow others to impose on you. Remember that the less-lauded motivations for a career in medicine often tend to be the weaker ones. Finally, take into account that medicine is changing, and some of your expectations—for salary, independence, or close physician-patient bonds—may become more difficult to realize.

REFERENCES

1. Heisenberg W: *Physics and Philosophy*. New York, Harper & Row, 1958, p 205.
2. Telephone interview with American Medical Association staff member, 23 January 1986. Quoted from Duran D, Reynolds R: *Social Economics Characteristics of Medical Practice*. Chicago, American Medical Association, 1985.
3. Relman AS: The future of medical practice. *Health Affairs* 2:13-18, 1983.
4. Marketing helps physician meet patient needs. *Mich Med* 83:168, 1984.

2

Laying the Groundwork in High School

"If I had eight hours to chop down a tree,
I'd spend six sharpening my ax."

ABRAHAM LINCOLN

WHAT YOU SHOULDN'T KNOW

I can still picture Alan Berman, at age 15, sitting in English class. He was talking about his future as an orthopedic surgeon, a doctor who specializes in operations on bones and tendons. Someone had told him that orthopedic surgeons often treat professional athletes, and Alan liked that idea. At the time, neither of us had watched surgery being performed, and we had no idea that orthopedic surgeons must train for six years after medical school, often sleeping over in the hospital every other night.

Alan was like many people who ultimately apply to medical school. He was well-organized, even slightly compulsive—the kind of person who disliked loose ends. His desire to categorize ideas and to quickly complete a task at hand extended beyond his research papers and homework assignments and influenced the way he thought and planned. But by jumping to completely define his career, Alan was playing at decision-making before he had all the necessary information.

As tempting as it might be to role-play during high school, it is a big enough step to express an interest in medicine and explore the profession in the few ways which we will discuss. Focusing in on a particular specialty is something with which third- and fourth-year students in medical school must grapple; it can only serve to limit unnecessarily your exposure at this early stage. These are years to appreciate the breadth of medicine.

WORKING AT A LOCAL HOSPITAL

One way to gain early exposure to medicine is by working at a nearby hospital. Many hospitals have formalized programs which carry with them a structured way of choosing volunteers;

19

some even utilize a lottery system to select from the many applicants for their few positions. The best of these programs are well-organized and periodically reviewed to ensure that students are receiving a worthwhile hospital experience. However, some programs lack adequate direction, and since they fall under the umbrella of the "volunteer office," they may be too structured to allow you to explore special interests or to spend extra time with one physician whose work you find particularly interesting.

One way to find out whether a particular program is likely to provide you with a good learning experience is by requesting the names of a few participants from the previous year. Past participants can give you personal perspectives on the positive and negative aspects of various hospital jobs. Keep in mind that their memories of the program may be flavored by prior expectations of, and by new insight into, the medical profession. If last year's emergency room worker decided that medicine was not for him, his memories of the hospital may be less than objective. Ask questions that call for direct answers: Did the participant feel that the doctors were accessible and willing to talk about medicine? Was all of his or her time taken by chores? Were volunteers allowed to watch medical or surgical procedures being performed? Having completed the program, does he or she know more about the medical profession?

After talking with past participants, make an honest effort to identify the conditions under which you work best. If you find meeting people easy and consider tight schedules a burden, then a less-structured experience may be best for you. On the other hand, if you feel you would like your day planned in advance, look for a program that makes clear where, when, and with whom you will be working.

Many formal programs include work in the emergency room as an orderly or patient advocate (a person who directs patients to appropriate areas and, hopefully, puts them at ease). Whether or not hospitals in your area have such specific employment programs for high school students, however, you may choose to try to structure a program of your own. One way is by personally contacting a physician on the staff of a nearby hospital. Ask to spend a month or two helping out in his or her office or watching the surgical procedures he or she performs.

Alternatively, you may design a role for yourself and offer a service to the physician or the hospital. If you would like the opportunity to watch surgery, for example, you could offer to transport patients from their hospital rooms to the operating room in exchange for clearance to watch procedures later in the day.

Most students meet with greater success when job hunting by offering their services as volunteers. You can certainly ask if any funding is available, but remember that the most important dividend of the time you spend working will be your insight into the medical profession. If earning spending money is a must, limit your hours at the hospital or physician's office to allow for another part-time job. Consider your volunteer hours an investment that can pay invaluable dividends if they lead to a more rational career decision.

Finally, don't expect that the time you spend working in a doctor's office or a hospital during high school will answer all of your questions about the profession. Unfortunately, it will be many years before you have a clear idea of what it is really like to practice medicine. Medicine is a diverse, complex, and changing field. My friends and I only began to appreciate it fully as we moved out of the classroom and onto the wards during the third year of medical school. You may be encouraged or discouraged after your initial exposure. Make a mental note about how the experience made you feel, but keep in mind that you still have very limited information.

SELECTING A COLLEGE

In the preface to this book I promised to tell you "what works"—what steps you can take to make your admission to medical school more likely. I promised to outline the best route to success at each step of the process, and I will. But I also want to caution you against stalking admission blindly and missing out on other important experiences.

Your college years can be four of the most intellectually satisfying and broadening years of your life. Moreover, they can be a tremendous amount of fun. If you choose correctly, your undergraduate school will provide you with even more important advantages than a good position from which to apply to medical school.

You should look first for a school that will take an interest in you as a person and that offers opportunities to explore diverse areas of study. Seek a college or university at which you believe you will feel comfortable for four years. Consider the size of the school, its strong and weak departments, its location, and the activism or apathy of the student body. Remember that you will be studying and socializing at your undergraduate school for four years—too long to compromise learning and enjoyment in the name of admission to graduate school.

If a small, lesser-known school seems like the place where you would be happiest, enroll there. My medical school class at Johns Hopkins is filled with graduates not only from Harvard and Yale, but from Dickinson College and Arizona State University. When you apply to medical school, the most important factors will be your personal achievements and level of interest, not your alma mater.

Since becoming a physician is one of the possibilities you are now considering, however, make certain that the college you attend offers the courses required for application to medical school. It may also be to your benefit if the school has a premedical advisory program to help you chart your way through premedical studies and the application process.

Having been cautioned against basing your choice of a college solely on the headstart it might give you toward medical school, you should be aware that there are indices you can use to assess whether a college will put you at any advantage or disadvantage should you decide to pursue a medical education.

One index is the college or university's track record. Inquire about the percentage of medical school applicants who were accepted over the past five years. The number of admissions alone is not helpful, of course; a school with five applicants and five admissions impresses me more than a school with 30 admissions and 300 applicants.

You should also ask for a rough estimate of what percentage of premedical students go on to apply to medical school. Some colleges have inflated rates of acceptance because they have designed their premedical curricula to weed out as many borderline applicants as possible before they get the chance to apply. If these figures are unavailable from the admissions office, you can get a sense of how much weeding out goes on by talking to premedical students. Just take some time to visit the library and ask questions.

Yet another consideration is whether the school has a medical school associated with it. This is important for two reasons. First, a nearby medical school and teaching hospital will give you access to summer positions in research and hospital care which you might otherwise find more difficult to obtain. Second, a medical school with an associated undergraduate school often accepts a disproportionate number of its own college's applicants—a welcome edge if you need an advantage when it comes time to apply.

Some universities with medical schools actually offer combined BA-MD programs. These continua offer the promise of almost-automatic admission to medical school when you are admitted as an undergraduate. There are costs, however, associated with such programs, and these will be discussed in the next section.

Finally, to end where we began, keep in mind that your college years can be a wonderful experience whether or not your school gets 90 percent of its applicants into medical school. Pick your college as a college, not as a stepping stone. If you decide not to enter the medical profession, you will want to be at a school that offers many other opportunities. If you do become a physician, you and the field will only benefit from the wide perspective you cultivated as an undergraduate.

COMBINED BA-MD PROGRAMS

Several colleges and universities offer combined undergraduate-medical school programs which students begin after high school (see Appendix). These continua last either six or seven years, but many can be extended to eight years if the enrolled student so desires. Typically, the student spends two or three years as an undergraduate and then begins the four years of medical school. There may be requirements to move into the medical school phase of the program, such as a "B" average or adequate performance on the Medical Colleges Admission Test.

Combined programs have existed since the 1950s. Some were created in an attempt to provide a more "liberal curriculum" by mixing courses in the humanities with those in the medical sciences. Others were created in response to a perceived shortage of physicians. Whatever the original intent of the programs, they call for a decision to enter medicine at the same time the student applies to college—Alan Berman's dream.

A 1961 study by the Association of American Medical Colleges (AAMC), recognizing the potential problems such programs could create, reflected, "How many people, having made an early commitment to medicine, will change their minds or, still worse, continue in a field of study where they really do not belong?" (1).

The AAMC's point is well taken. As we have already discussed, it is nearly impossible to make an informed career decision as a junior or senior in high school. An educational program that asks you to do just that should arouse your suspicion.

Administrators associated with one of the accelerated medical programs, in fact, explained to me that part of the underlying intent of the BA-MD was actually to attract better students to their campus. The academic credentials of applicants to the combined program at this university are far more impressive than those of students who apply to the university's medical school at the end of college. "The program uses a carrot of early admission to medical school to lure top students—students who would otherwise end up at Harvard Medical School and the like. We'd never get them to apply later on," one dean said.

If you are swayed by the early admission offer, there are important questions you should ask before signing on. First, inquire whether you will have the option of expanding the program to eight years if you feel you need more time to get a sufficiently broad education. Second, ask whether you will forfeit your reserved seat in the university's medical school by applying to other schools of medicine after your undergraduate training—by applying "outside." If there is no option to extend the program to eight years and no provision for outside application, seriously consider whether you are locking yourself into a program that may not offer you what you want in six months, or a year, or two years.

Here, again, I urge you not to select a college simply because it offers an accelerated medical program. Evaluate the college as a college, and, as always, ask students enrolled in the program for their impressions. Should you enter a combined degree program, you will be spending a great deal of time with the other BA-MD students. Make sure they seem like a group you will be able to tolerate.

LETTING CURIOSITY AND CONFIDENCE
BE YOUR GUIDES

One of my college roommates at Brown told me that when he was in the tenth grade he had contacted medical schools to express his interest in medicine. At that time, he was already considering a number of career paths and was anxious to explore each on a limited basis. Far from thinking him too forward, several medical school administrators invited him to tour their schools' facilities and offered him advice as he began to learn about the profession. He acted on his strong curiosity about medicine and was rewarded with early contact with the medical school environment.

Throughout the process of preparing for and applying to medical school, allow your curiosity and your self-confidence to direct you. You should act on your interest in any way in which you feel comfortable. Simply because there are traditional routes and traditional times to explore professions doesn't mean that your own novel approach won't meet with equal or greater success.

Keep in mind, however, that curiosity and confidence, not the fear of being left behind, are the best guides. Learning about the medical profession is not a race, and there will be time to explore later on if your level of interest has not yet peaked.

REFERENCES

1. Severinghaus AE, et. al.: *Preparation for Medical Education: A Restudy.* New York, McGraw-Hill, 1961.

3

Premedical Education

"Men are men before they are lawyers
or physicians or manufacturers;
and, if you make them capable and
sensible men, they will make themselves
capable and sensible lawyers
and physicians."

JOHN STUART MILL

REQUIREMENTS FOR ADMISSION
TO MEDICAL SCHOOL

Welcome to the world of investment. The currency you will use will not be dollars and cents, but time and effort. Premedical students often use the words "delayed gratification" to express the fact that many of the courses they must complete and excel in are not of special interest to them, but, simply, pieces of the curriculum vitae for acceptance to medical school—a "means to an end." They often remind themselves, as you should, that studying organic chemistry and physics does not resemble practicing medicine. Your level of excitement at the synthetic pathway of buna-S-rubber is no measure of your potential as a physician.

Whether or not you are enamored of the requirements for admission to medical school, you must know what the requirements are at the various schools to which you will be applying. One of the medical students I live with found himself scrambling to schedule calculus during his fourth year of college after he realized, late in the game, that Johns Hopkins requires the course. He was able to complete it in time, but the extra course hours made his senior year rockier than it needed to be.

The basic premedical curriculum includes one year each of biology (with lab), general chemistry (with lab), organic chemistry (with lab), and physics (with lab). Individual schools frequently require a year of English and a year of mathematics (some specifying completion of calculus) as well. Some schools, in fact, insist on or strongly recommend other courses ranging from psychology to biochemistry.

Many medical schools report requiring only three years of undergraduate education. Completing a four-year degree program, however, can only strengthen an applicant's academic record. Plan to enjoy your senior year of college before beginning professional training.

While the final selection of medical schools to which you will apply will take place during your junior year, it is wise, early on in college, to identify and investigate several schools that are of special interest to you. These might include medical schools in your home state, the school associated with your college, the schools from which your relatives graduated, and schools that, for any reason, you see as particularly attractive.

You will find much of the information you need in *Medical School Admission Requirements*, a yearly publication of the Association of American Medical Colleges (AAMC) that lists the specific admissions requirements of all accredited medical schools in the United States. Order a copy (current price is $7.50 shipped book rate) and make sure that you schedule time during college to fulfill the special requirements of schools on your early preference list. *Medical School Admission Requirements* can be ordered from:

> Association of American Medical Colleges
> Attn: Membership and Publication Orders
> Suite 200, One Dupont Circle, NW
> Washington, D.C. 20036

It is also useful to obtain catalogues from each of the medical schools on your list. Medical school addresses are included in the AAMC publication. You should send a postcard requesting a catalogue to the admissions office of each of the schools on your list.

YOUR COLLEGE MAJOR

Undergraduate students must choose a "major"—an area of concentrated study in which they will earn a degree. It is generally not possible to major in "premed." Being "premed" simply means that you plan to complete the requirements we have talked about and to apply to medical school.

For decades, many physicians and educators have called for more "liberal" premedical education. They have voiced their objections to narrowly-focused undergraduate study over and over again in reports published by the AAMC. In 1953, a study of premedical education in the United States concluded:

> Two stumbling blocks in the way of liberalizing premedical education would be removed if all medical school officers would declare their support of a more liberal education as a preparation for medical students, and if premedical advisors would stop questioning the sincerity of their declarations (1).

In the 1980s, it is clear that majoring in a nonscience, far from weakening your application, will serve you well when you apply to medical school. The breadth of your undergraduate education and your ability to master subjects other than basic sciences will be seen as assets that will allow you to enrich the experience of your classmates and to relate effectively to your future patients.

You should feel free to concentrate in any area of interest to you. A high percentage of applicants still choose to major in biology or chemistry (some of the required courses for these majors overlap with requirements for admission to medical school), and, if either appeals to you, there is certainly no reason to avoid pursuing that field. But there is also no reason to avoid in-depth study of East Asian history, and such an unusual base of knowledge might even be attractive to admissions committees.

The field of medicine itself will require more and more physicians with diverse backgrounds as continuing challenges in economics, public policy, and public health call for medical professionals who can understand complex problems.

The most important reason to pursue your own interests in college is, however, your own enlightenment. Your college years are a unique time. You will have close at hand many talented students and dedicated teachers creating a wonderful environment in which to learn. An area of study that you find enjoyable and that sustains your curiosity will not only be an adequate preparation for medical school, but a valuable training ground for intellectual skills that will serve you well throughout life.

RATIONAL COURSE SELECTION

If everyone involved in the medical school admissions process could be relied upon to assess each of your grades critically and give proper weight to the difficulty of each course, then rational course selection would simply mean signing up for whichever and however many courses seem interesting. A "C" in Professor Sadism's backbreaking comparative anatomy class would bring the same rave reviews as an "A" in a less demanding chemistry class. Everyone would understand how hard it is just to pass Sadism's course.

Forget it. In the real world only other students at your school will know about Professor Sadism's four-hour tests—admissions committees almost certainly will not. The courses you and your classmates recognize as incredibly easy (a "B" for writing your name correctly on the midterm) and incredibly difficult (an "A" for being the most talented student ever to enroll in the course) will be computer-printed course titles on your transcript.

If getting into medical school is one of your primary goals, you will have to be able to make a critical assessment of your abilities and avoid getting low grades in infamous courses. If your college has a pass/fail option, consider electing not to receive a letter grade in a particularly difficult course which, nonetheless, interests you. Alternatively, you may choose to save that upper-level mammalian neuroendocrine physiology course for a particularly light semester or for the second semester of your senior year when you may already have been accepted by the medical school of your choice.

Choosing courses that are both interesting and less difficult can lighten the load during a semester that may include other extremely challenging classes. A course that is particularly appealing to you, in fact, even if it requires a bit more time, can depressurize your premedical years by bringing your other interests and skills into play. Take studio art or a course in 19th century poetry. Vagabond through as many departments as you like. Don't stop at getting into medical school; get educated.

Just as it is sometimes wise to opt out of elective courses that would probably result in a lower grade than you want on your transcript, it is possible to take premedical requirements at schools other than your own college. A few of my classmates at Brown took physics courses during the summer at less competitive universities close to their homes. If you know that your school's organic chemistry class, for example, is poorly organized or unusually difficult, consider taking it elsewhere. Make sure, however, that the course at another college will be an adequate introduction to the particular topic it addresses. You may decide, next semester or next year, to take a course that builds on the foundation it was supposed to provide. Also, be sure that the course you sign up for at another school is actually less strenuous. Small, innocuous-looking colleges often pride themselves on the rigorous educational path trodded by their graduates.

A few students elect to take an extra course during one or two semesters of their undergraduate education. Picking up the pace in this way should be done cautiously. Not only does a fifth course (at a school where the norm is four courses per semester) translate to a 25 percent greater load, but it will also take time away from extracurricular activities which might teach you more in a less formal setting. An extra course can also seriously limit your relaxation time. I learned as much propped against pillows in my dorm room discussing religion and politics with my hallmates as I did in some of my classes.

Keep in mind that much of rational course selection hinges on honestly assessing your own abilities. If taking five courses that include an upper-level neurophysiology class doesn't cramp your style, then feel free to schedule them. Learn as much as you can without losing sleep.

Finally, many premedical students are tempted to take college courses that will be given, at a more rapid pace, in medical school. They enroll in anatomy, biochemistry, microbiology, and the like in order to make the first year of medical school less difficult. To a limited extent, these expectations are valid. Taking biochemistry at Brown made the course somewhat easier for me at Johns Hopkins. At one time during my first year of medical school, I was also glad that I had taken neural science as an undergraduate. The bottom line, however, is that students arrive at medical school with varied backgrounds. Many have knowledge about one or two subjects before the courses begin, but even those who have taken the bare minimum of premedical requirements make it through. A course taken in preparation for medical school should never replace the writing course you always hoped to take or the drama class everyone has been talking about. You will be in medical school for four years and will probably yearn for the diversity of undergraduate education at least once or twice. Enjoy that diversity now.

YOUR PREMEDICAL ADVISOR

There is no mandatory training for premedical advisors. Most are not physicians themselves, and their insights into the medical school admissions process vary greatly. There will generally be a consensus of sorts among juniors and seniors as to whether or not your college's advisor has been helpful and well-informed. Ask for their impressions and take their opinions seriously. If your premedical advisor has been of great help to your predecessors, you can probably rely on him or her to provide accurate and up-to-date information. If, however, there is general dissatisfaction with the advisor's perceived level of competence, "adopt" another advisor. A particularly talented premedical advisor will often be willing to spend time with students from other colleges, and informal advice may also be obtained from professors at a nearby medical school.

Even if you find that your college's premedical advisor is not to be relied upon, it is important that this person gain an appreciation of your commitment to medicine and your interests and talents. This is not "brown-nosing" (appearing friendly and interested just to capture the support of those with influence over your future), but, rather, it is assuring that your advisor has sufficient information to assist you. He or she will be expected, either with a committee or alone, to evaluate you in a letter to the medical schools to which you apply. This letter may be separate from, or a composite of, the recommendations you will obtain from professors or other physicians with whom you have worked. The contents of this letter have a clear impact on your success as an applicant, and the first time you speak at length with your advisor should not be at the last minute—as the application deadline approaches. Your interests and his or her competency as your advocate will both be served if you make early contact during freshman year and stay in touch as you move through the premedical curriculum. It is not necessary that you report a firm commitment to attending medical school; expressing an interest is enough to begin the relationship. Be open and involve your advisor in your evolving career decisions.

The bottom line, even if juniors and seniors give your premedical advisor rave reviews, is that you should devote some of your own time to becoming knowledgeable about the application process. A valuable source of information for applicants is *The Advisor*, a newsletter for premedical advisors which helps to keep them informed. Another worthwhile publication is the *Journal of Medical Education* which gives an annual profile of the year's successful medical school applicants, including their average GPA's (grade point averages), MCAT (Medical College Admission Test) scores, etc. JAMA (the *Journal of the American*

Medical Association) publishes an annual issue on medical education which contains statistics that can also help you to become an informed applicant.

CULTIVATING STUDENT-FACULTY RELATIONSHIPS

The best reason to establish close relationships with faculty members is that their age and experience can offer you life perspectives that are impossible to obtain from your peers. Your own curiosity should lead you to tap the resource that professors represent and to establish friendships with those few instructors with whom you feel a special affinity. The fact that some of these teachers may ultimately be called upon to recommend you for admission to medical school in no way diminishes the worth or honesty of your interaction with them. They become the logical evaluators of you as a person and future professional because they know you best.

Many students find it difficult to begin such relationships because they seem to be outside the standard student-faculty rapport. Nothing could be further from the truth. Professors have chosen formal education as their stock in trade for a variety of reasons, but many particularly enjoy their potential role as sculptors of the next generation of scholars and teachers. By going to a professor with questions not only about yesterday's assignment or tomorrow's exam, but also with broader concerns about his field of interest or your response to it, you will enrich your undergraduate experience and provide a potential evaluator with information about you as a person.

Just as it makes little sense for your interaction with a premedical advisor to begin at the time when you are ready to apply to medical school, your relationships with faculty members can start during your first semester of college. A trusted faculty member-friend can be one of the most worthwhile rewards of your undergraduate education. Such relationships also, of course, lead to stronger recommendations—not because you have "brown-nosed," but because you have cultivated real and lasting interpersonal bonds.

SUMMER JOBS

Many of the positions we talked about in Chapters 1 and 2 need simply to be echoed here. "Shadowing" a physician or working as a volunteer in a hospital will certainly provide you with additional career information during college, and your background in the sciences, however limited, may make you a more attractive applicant for hospital jobs.

The summers of your college years are also appropriate periods for participation in research. Research, yet another opportunity in medicine, includes clinical research with patients and basic science research in the lab. You may want to experience either or both of these. Projects that you begin during the summer, especially if connected with a hospital or medical school near your college, can often be continued in your spare time during the academic year.

Some medical schools tend to look with particular favor on applicants who have demonstrated even a minor interest in medical research. No school will fault you for having explored the area. Participating for a short period of time will also allow you to select more accurately the medical schools to which you will apply—certain institutions stress the importance of medi-cal research and attract students interested in making it part of their careers.

Certainly, the hospital wards or laboratories are not the only places where human efforts translate to societal gain. Medical school admissions committees are also likely to be favorably impressed by work with the handicapped, with social service organizations, or in public health. Your own interests should dictate what kind of summer or extracurricular work you do. The current awareness that medicine can only benefit from students with a diversity of experience makes your range of choices quite broad.

While many students find work in a hospital or lab through friends of the family or undergraduate professors, a limited listing of many such opportunities may be found in the annual directory of internships published by Writer's Digest Books. Many libraries have the most current volume in their reference sections. I used *1983 Internships* to investigate summer positions to follow my first year of medical school.

Again, many of the available positions are nonsalaried. As was necessary during high school, you may need to limit the hours or number of weeks you spend as a volunteer in order to earn money. Remember that a volunteer experience that provides information about the medical profession or one that positions you well for admission to medical school is worth the time you invest.

EXTRACURRICULAR ACTIVITIES
DURING THE ACADEMIC YEAR

Medical schools seem especially enamored of late with the well-rounded applicant. They smile upon those who appear not only to have coped with the demands of premedical education, but also to have demonstrated a commitment to outside interests, real personal growth, and campus or community groups.

The traditional premedical extracurricular activities, including work in a hospital or research laboratory, remain important. Such positions, which we have discussed as possible summer experiences, are relatively easy ways to find out more about the medical profession and to demonstrate interest in the field. Neither of the two is essential for successful application to medical school, but without this work your understanding of, and commitment to, the profession may seem less well-grounded.

While some exposure to research or clinical care outside the classroom is desirable, it is not sufficient. The most successful applicant will have used his or her time to pursue a special interest and will have achieved a position of leadership in that area. Working through the ranks of your student government and accepting increasing responsibility will be viewed more favorably than dabbling in six different campus groups.

While an applicant's special interest may, in fact, be a particular project in medical research, the current emphasis on diversity in premedical education makes it possible, even beneficial, to use extracurricular time to learn about a nonscientific field. My housemate trained as a clown during college and entertained professionally before being admitted to Hopkins. He had also volunteered in a hospital, but I think you can guess which activity generated more discussion at the admissions committee meeting.

Certain bases have to be covered, but pursuing your own interests is, fortunately, the best game plan. Identifying areas of special interest, related or unrelated to medicine, and making significant contributions on or off campus are more than the stuff of which good applications are made; they're what college is all about.

"PREMED SYNDROME" AND MAINTAINING BALANCE

Investments, particularly risky ones, are usually made by the entrepreneurial spirits among us whose nature it is to take chances and hope for large returns. By investing the bulk of his or her undergraduate years preparing for application to medical school, however, the relatively conservative premedical student is also taking a risk. Many students live with substantial uncertainty about their chances for acceptance to medical school, and even the brightest students seem never to be completely convinced that failure isn't lurking in next semester's organic chemistry class or disguising itself as the Medical College Admission Test.

The tension is understandable. Approximately half the applicants who seek admission to medical school are not accepted (2). This, together with the fact that the premedical curriculum may prepare the applicant only for medical school, means that premedical students run the risk of finding themselves unaccepted by their chosen profession and unmarketable in any other profession following college graduation. Not so for prelaw students who require no special courses for admission to graduate school and may comfortably establish a valuable background in business administration, marketing, or engineering.

The response of the premedical student is often to over-compensate for this tenuous position by throwing himself or herself headlong into studies, excluding other interests, social life, and development as a person. "Take no chances" becomes the undergraduate motto and leads to Friday and Saturday nights in the library and alarm clocks set to 7 a.m. on Sunday mornings. You may already have in your mind a stereotyped image of the student suffering from premedical syndrome. He or she isn't seen at parties, hasn't joined a fraternity or sorority because the house might be too noisy, avoids literature and history courses for fear of "B's," is the first to arrive at the library, and the last to leave—gaunt, exhausted, and ready for more work back at the dorm.

Some of the uglier byproducts of premedical syndrome are academic dishonesty and real psychological impairment. More-over, obvious victims of the syndrome are outnumbered by the hard-to-diagnose sufferers whose anxiety and depressed mood remain hidden in the cafeteria or in the dormitory, but sur-face during private calls home.

There are several ways to prevent premedical syndrome from making your undergraduate education intolerable. First, you should realize that the germ that causes this disease is not within you, but within the educational system. Feeling stress and responding by turning inward and working as hard as pos-sible is a foreseeable reaction that could occur in anyone faced with the demands and uncertainties of premedical education. The lack of support systems at colleges adds to the problem. There is no inherent weakness in you reflected by a rocky road during premedical study. Keeping that fact in mind should help you to externalize some of the stress you may experience and to maintain perspective.

You should also remember that you are not the only student feeling "stressed out" by premedical requirements and the desire to attend medical school. "Premed syndrome" is common, even among those whose tough exteriors hide their frustrations and anxieties. It is often helpful to talk openly about your concerns with other students, with an accessible professor, or with your premedical advisor. There may be little they can do to alleviate the stressors inherent in organic chemistry and the MCAT, but they can often suggest study habits or social habits to ease the load.

There are a few simple steps that premedical students can take to prevent or recover from premedical syndrome. Alloting a given period of time—perhaps Friday evening after dinner and Sunday morning until noon—as free time can make the rest of the week more livable. You may also decide to spend one full hour at dinner each night, no matter how many chemistry problems are due the next day. This reserved time should not be compromised for anything short of an impending final exam (if that). This will be your time to socialize, read a novel, or go for a walk without feeling guilty that you are not in the library studying. You should view it as untouchable "mental health time." Allowing yourself to have this time will only enhance your performance on assignments. Clearing your mind now and then will make academic achievement easier.

Another way to stay healthy is by building a world outside premedical studies so that you can maintain balance. Extracurricular activities and nonscience course work can help, as can consciously making friends interested in careers other than medicine. Like the prelaw student, you may find it worthwhile to structure activities and courses that actually prepare you in some way for an alternative career. Working as editor of the *Brown Banner* and taking courses in literature, persuasive writing, and journalism reminded me that another pathway (journalism) was open should my interest in medicine dwindle or my road to medical school acceptance be blocked. Even beyond this "safety valve" function, work outside the premedical curriculum is simply part of taking full advantage of your college years. You owe it to yourself.

It is important that you not abandon outside interests when your college years begin. If you followed politics closely in high school, bring a copy of the city newspaper to the library with you and read it for a half hour before you read your physics textbook. Take a course in international relations. Read 15 pages of *Democracy in America* (3) before bed each night. Stay whole.

As you move further into the premedical years you will be increasingly able to assess your chances for acceptance to medical school. If your level of achievement is high enough that you feel relatively confident about admission, you will probably automatically branch further into areas of special interest to you and leave the premedical syndrome behind. Do not be afraid to ask your premedical advisor where you stand relative to those students who typically gain admission from your college. The information he or she provides can help you to set a rational pace. You may find it possible to achieve the same grades with fewer nights in the library.

If premedical education remains a constant struggle for you, your investment will be greater than average. Even though you already know that premed courses tell you nothing about whether you will enjoy practicing medicine, you will have to give serious consideration to whether you are willing to make the enormous sacrifices that are unavoidable not only during college, but also during medical school. Things get harder, and eight years of stress may simply not be worth it to you.

But it might. Do not confuse the premedical syndrome with commitment. If achieving the goal of becoming a doctor is important to you, and if you are among those who must make particularly substantial sacrifices to reach that goal, never be embarassed by your efforts. Staying in the library on Saturday nights might be the only way you can keep the possibility of attending medical school feasible. True friends will understand and respect your ambition and discipline.

The best news is that with all the hurdles encountered during premedical education, not only can you make it through, but you can enjoy four years of unusual personal growth. Guarding your personal interests and maintaining a sense of perspective about your work are the keys to your success.

REFERENCES

1. Severinghaus AE, et. al.: *Preparation for Medical Education in a Liberal Arts College.* New York, McGraw-Hill, 1953.

2. Association of American Medical Colleges: *Medical School Admission Requirements 1985-1986.* Washington, D.C., AAMC, 1984, p 10.

3. De Tocqueville A: *Democracy in America.* New York, New American Library, 1956.

4

The Medical College Admission Test (MCAT)

"Nothing in education is so astonishing as the amount of ignorance it accumulates in the form of inert facts" (1).

HENRY BROOKS ADAMS

WHY THE MCAT EXISTS

Since students apply to medical school from colleges that have curricula with vastly different levels of difficulty, medical school admissions committees are faced with the task of comparing applicants whose grades may not fairly reflect their levels of achievement. As we have already discussed, a reliable weighting system that would make a "B-" from Yale University equal an "A" from Easystreet College does not exist. Medical schools have traditionally clung to MCAT scores as a method of more objectively ranking applicants and predicting the likelihood of their success as medical students. The Association of American Medical Colleges (AAMC), which administers the MCAT, also maintains that the exam has been designed so that a given score in 1986 will reflect the same level of accomplishment as that score in 1990, allowing comparison between applicants who have taken the test at different times.

What the MCAT actually measures is at best unclear. The AAMC, in its booklet *The MCAT Student Manual* (2), states that subsections of the MCAT have been designed to "assess your understanding of concepts and principles in science that have been identified as important prerequisites for the study of medicine." Many medical educators, however, question whether the MCAT actually predicts success in medical school and seriously doubt that it is at all useful in predicting who will be a good doctor. In 1985, The Johns Hopkins University School of Medicine eliminated the MCAT as an admission requirement.

Indeed, the AAMC's own panel on physician education, the Panel on the General Professional Education of the Physician and College Preparation for Medicine (GPEP), concluded in its report, *Physicians for the Twenty-First Century* (3), that MCAT scores are often overemphasized in evaluating applicants. The MCAT is designed to assess, the report states, "only part of the students' overall qualifications to study medicine." You, yourself, in reviewing for the test, should remember that its use of multiple-choice questions is too superficial and its focus on biology, chemistry, and physics is too narrow. Your study of history and literature, your facility at putting people at ease, and, certainly, your writing ability are also important parts of your preparation to study and to practice medicine.

HOW IMPORTANT IS THE TEST?

Academic institutions change slowly. For the foreseeable future, the MCAT will remain a major measure by which applicants are evaluated, and many medical schools with narrow views of physician education will continue to overemphasize your scores. Because the weight the MCAT carries will vary with each admissions committee, you must assume that it may be assigned as much importance as your grade point average. It is essential, therefore, to take the MCAT seriously and to prepare well for it.

By preparing extensively for the MCAT, you can use the MCAT to your advantage. The MCAT is an opportunity to demonstrate competency (at least what will be perceived as competency) in the academic areas generally covered during premedical education. The MCAT can, therefore, be a second chance for students who feel that their grades reflect less than they have learned and an equalizer for students from lesser-known colleges. Even for premedical students with excellent grades from well-known institutions, the MCAT is a chance to distinguish themselves from the crowd and gain acceptance to top schools.

The fact that a single test could seriously impact on one's chances for admission to medical school looms ominously in the back of the premedical mind. Anxiety sets in many months before the exam is given. Students begin to wonder whether they have actually retained all the equations from chemistry and concepts from physics which they were taught.

The best way to keep MCAT anxiety under control is to begin preparing for the test early and to do a thorough job of it. Knowing that you are well-prepared will allow you to feel more relaxed during your junior year, and the confidence that comes with excellent preparation may even translate to higher scores on exam day.

WHAT TO EXPECT

Expect a long day. The MCAT is divided into four main parts; actual time for working on the test is 6½ hours. The first part, given during the morning of the test day, is the Science Knowledge Subtest (135 minutes) which is composed of 125 questions further divided into three subsections—biology, chemistry, and physics. The questions are multiple choice, and those in each subsection test your knowledge of that specific field only.

After a short rest period, the MCAT continues with the Science Problems Subtest. These 66 multiple-choice questions are presented in groups of three, each group based on a short descriptive passage which may contain irrelevant information or data that must be reworked. Problems may require that you bring into play knowledge of different areas in biology, chemistry, and physics. This section of the MCAT tends to be the most challenging.

The MCAT essay currently completes the morning session. Students read a short passage and respond to a question based on its content. The essay is an experimental addition to the MCAT; the AAMC has not yet decided whether it will become a permanent part of the exam. Medical school admissions committees will have access to the essays of applicants to the 1987 entering class, but it is not known how much weight the essay will carry in the admissions process or even how it will be evaluated.

The final two parts of the MCAT, the Skills Analysis Subtests, are given after lunch. The Reading Subtest and Quantitative Subtest, separated by a short break, are each composed of 68 questions. Multiple-choice questions follow a reading selection or a set of data, respectively.

Since your scores will be determined by the number of questions you answer correctly, you should answer every question, guessing at those of which you are unsure. Questions left blank will be counted the same as questions answered incorrectly. That means that there is no penalty for guessing and no excuse for not filling in a letter for every multiple-choice question. Blindly guessing on a question with five possible answers gives you a 20 percent chance of being right.

The four subtests of the MCAT are used to generate six different scores: (1) Biology Knowledge, (2) Chemistry Knowledge, (3) Physics Knowledge, (4) Science Problems, (5) Skills Analysis: Reading, and (6) Skills Analysis: Quantitative.

The Science Problems portion of the MCAT actually counts twice—it influences each Science Knowledge score and is also reported as a separate score.

Your test results will be reported on a scale of 1 (worst) to 15 (best). A 15-point scale means that slight differences in the performance of students will be minimized. It's bad enough that some medical schools might rank applicants with 10s differently than those with 11s. Imagine if they were allowed to split hairs between 36 correct answers versus 37.

GETTING READY: REGISTERING AND PREPARING FOR THE MCAT

The MCAT is given each year in April and again in September. You should register for the spring testing date during your junior year. The only legitimate reason to sign up for the fall test is not having completed essential background courses which you have scheduled for the summer. Waiting until the fall exam will delay your scores until winter, and your chances of early interviews and acceptances will be greatly reduced. Some medical schools, in fact, do not accept the fall test results for application in that calendar year. Taking the MCAT during April will also allow you to retake the exam, if necessary, in time for medical schools to glance at your second scores.

You can register for the MCAT beginning in February. Registration packets are often available from your premedical advisor, but can also be obtained by writing directly to:

MCAT Registration
American College Testing Program
P.O. Box 414
Iowa City, IA 52240

Passport photos (2" X 2") are required for the MCAT and will also be needed for many of your medical school applications. Purchase approximately 15 copies to have on hand.

Registering for the MCAT and taking it are the easy parts. The bulk of your energy will be expended in preparation for the test. To begin, you should order a copy of *The MCAT Student Manual* and *The Practice Medical College Admission Test* (4) and work through the multiple choice items in each. The manual not only contains sample problems, but also explains the various types of questions on the MCAT and gives a general outline of what each subtest covers. Both can be ordered from:

Association of American Medical Colleges
Attention: Membership and Publication Orders
One Dupont Circle, NW
Washington, DC 20036

What should happen next is controversial. Everyone agrees that you should begin preparing early, spending a small amount of time each day for three or four months. There is considerable debate, however, about whether this time should be spent independently reviewing your course notes and textbooks or as a student in a commercial preparatory course, such as Stanley H. Kaplan (Stanley H. Kaplan Educational Centers, New York, New York). My own bias lies with signing on with one of the leading commercial courses. By presenting you with organized review materials and making available many sample tests, such courses allow you to make full use of your review time and to chart your progress as you move through the battery of mock exams.

Making proper use of a programmed review course means devoting time to the materials it provides. Stanley Kaplan won't do the work for you—signing up for his, or any other, course is useless if you aren't ready to make a commitment to preparing for the MCAT. Following through is the best way to minimize anxiety.

Another factor to consider is the price tag associated with a leading preparatory course. Many run over $400. You will have to assess whether you can afford to enroll. Though not well-advertised (for obvious reasons), some testing centers do offer reduced rates to students with demonstrable financial need. Others offer a less expensive package which includes renting study booklets and using taped materials without attending class. Ask about all the options.

On the other hand, there are certainly applicants who take no preparatory class and do very well on the MCAT. In fact, there is no real evidence that commercially prepared students fare significantly better than their independently prepared colleagues. What prep courses offer is a tranquilizer—a programmed review that relieves the student of the responsibility of deciding which material to study. If your scores on the Scholastic Aptitude Test (SAT) indicated your proficiency in taking standardized tests, if you feel well-prepared by your premedical coursework, and if you believe that you can muster the discipline to review adequately with class notes and textbooks, feel free to do so.

Finally, do not make late-night cramming sessions part of your strategy as the MCAT approaches. Getting enough sleep is more important than the few facts you might inhale from midnight to 2 a.m. You can't cram for a test that covers the entire premedical curriculum. Start early, and you will feel much more relaxed as April approaches.

WHEN TO BE SATISFIED

The MCAT can be taken again. Remember, though, taking a standardized test a second time doesn't ensure a higher score. You may do worse. In spite of the risk, a leading premedical advisor suggests that you should consider retaking the MCAT when you are three digits away from all nines. In other words:

One score of 8: Ignore

Two scores of 8: Borderline

Three scores of 8: Retake $[(9-8)\times3=3]$

One score of 8 and one score of 7:
   Retake $(9-8)+(9-7)=3]$

This is not a hard-and-fast rule, and you should not make the decision to retake the MCAT alone. Whether to retake the MCAT because of a score of seven on just one subtest, for example, is controversial. Ask your premedical advisor's opinion. Depending on your academic record, your premedical advisor may feel that a low score will receive less emphasis in your case or that your borderline performance will have to be improved. Share with your advisor any circumstance peculiar to the day you took the exam. Were you sick? Did you misread directions? Did you pace yourself poorly and not finish a subtest?

If you decide to retake the MCAT, prepare even more vigorously for the next testing date. If you did poorly in a single area, you will still need to review all others. Boosting your score in chemistry and lowering your score in biology is hardly a desirable outcome.

Whatever your scores, keep in mind that they reflect only one type of knowledge and should not be interpreted as a commentary on the kind of doctor you can become. What you did when you weren't studying for the MCAT would probably tell an admissions committee a lot more about that.

REFERENCES

1. Bartlett J: *Bartlett's Familiar Quotations.* Boston, Little, Brown and Company, 1968, p 777 as quoted from *The Education of Henry Adams,* Chapter 25.

2. Association of American Medical Colleges: *The MCAT Student Manual.* Washington, D.C., AAMC, 1984.

3. Association of American Medical Colleges: *Physician for the Twenty-First Century.* Washington, D.C., AAMC, 1984.

4. Association of American Medical Colleges: *The Practice Medical College Admission Test.* Washington, D.C., AAMC, 1984.

5

Applying to Medical School

"Keep away from people who try to belittle your ambition. Small people always do that, but the really great make you feel that you, too, can become great."

MARK TWAIN

ASSESSING YOUR CHANCES FOR ADMISSION

Having come this far, with years of long nights already invested and organic chemistry a blur, the temptation to play the admissions game reflexively is great. Even premedical students with relatively low grades and scores, if they have survived to this point, are eager for the delayed gratification we talked about.

The fact is that there is no GPA or MCAT cutoff below which admission to medical school is impossible. The idiosyncracies of the admissions processes at various medical schools combined with the unique academic and personal background of each applicant make it impossible to predict with 100 percent accuracy which students stand no chance of acceptance to medical school. According to AAMC figures, one 1984 applicant was even admitted with a GPA below 2.00 (below "C") (1). However, with the cost of applying to medical school sometimes topping $1500, it is important to make a critical assessment of your own chances. Students who recognize that their grades and scores are below average and who, nonetheless, want to make the investment in time and dollars will need to apply to a carefully selected group of schools and, probably, to a larger number of schools.

Your premedical advisor should be able to give you a sense of whether applicants with your credentials have met with success when applying to medical school. Schedule time with him or her and ask for an honest appraisal of your chances. If you still have questions, medical school admissions officers may be willing to comment informally on your record. Make the effort to ask their opinions. In addition, each year's *Medical School Admissions Requirements* generally contains a chart detailing the number of successful applicants with any given combination of grades and scores. You can use this table to get a very rough estimate of your chances of acceptance. The latest figures indicate that students with GPAs less than 3.0 find it particularly difficult to gain admission.

Regardless of what the charts, your advisor, and your friends say, no one who desires a career in medicine, who is willing to pay the price to apply (in dollars and hours), and who believes there is even a slight chance of his or her being accepted should be discouraged to the point of giving up. However, if your grades and scores are clearly below average, make backup plans for the year following graduation. Don't sit out the interviewing season for industry jobs if your acceptance to medical school is looking like "a real long shot."

TIME MANAGEMENT

Applying to medical school means more than writing a single essay and answering questions about your undergraduate course or study. Some schools will request that you write on specific topics, making it necessary for you to compose different essays for different applications. If you are fortunate enough to be offered interviews with several schools, you will want to, or may be required to, visit their facilities. Added to this is the time needed to tie loose ends—to make sure that scores and transcripts are sent well before deadlines and that faculty recommendations are returned on time to your premedical advisor.

Although medical schools report application deadlines from November to February (with few after December) of the year before enrollment, completing your applications during the summer following junior year will make your senior year much more relaxed and may actually increase your chances for admission. Each week, schedule some time away from part-time jobs and devote this time to getting applications ready for submission. The best strategy is to set up a schedule that commits you to completing a certain number of applications per week from June through August.

Professors generally understand that applicants to medical

school may sometimes miss classes during the fall or winter in order to be interviewed for medical school admission. When you schedule a visit to a medical school, share with each of your instructors the dates you will be away. Examinations may have to be rescheduled or deadlines extended. With careful planning, however, there is no reason for your academic performance to suffer. Remember that medical schools may receive your grades from senior year before a final decision on your application has been made.

SELECTING MEDICAL SCHOOLS

AAMC figures indicate that the average student applies to nine medical schools (1). There are significant numbers of applicants at either extreme, with some actually submitting only one application and others sending off well over 20.

With all the effort you have expended to reach this point, the application process is no time to scrimp and no time to take risks. If your credentials and your advisor make you confident of admission, you may apply to fewer schools than the borderline applicant, but even students with top grades and scores should apply to between five and 10 medical schools. Those with a reasonably good chance of admission should consider sending off between 10 and 15 applications, while applicants with questionable credentials would do well to submit between 15 and 20 applications. Whether or not you receive an acceptance letter, you'll know you've given the process your best shot.

The range of schools to which you apply is also important. Admission is far more competitive to some medical schools than to others, and even top candidates should select a spectrum of schools, from least selective to most selective, to which to apply. Since no one can be confident of admission to Harvard or Yale, your laundry list should include your top choices, a second group of intermediate choices, and a few relative "safeties"—schools where you and your premedical advisor feel you have an excellent chance of admission. If you have less glowing credentials, of course, you should limit yourself largely to less competitive programs. Keep in mind that there is no such thing as a "bad" medical school. What you take away from a school depends more on your commitment than on its reputation or resources.

State medical schools deserve special mention since they accept a large number of in-state residents. Other private institutions within your home state may receive public funding and have a commitment to admit a certain percentage of "in-staters," as well. You may have the best chance of admission at one of these schools, and you should seriously consider applying. The flip side is that some state schools accept very few or no out-of-state applicants. These schools are listed in the AAMC book and should almost always be avoided by the "out-of-stater."

Students from Alabama, Alaska, Idaho, Montana, Washington, and Wyoming should inquire with their premedical advisors about interstate agreements. Agreements, such as the Western Interstate Commission for Higher Education (WICHE) program, extend benefits normally reserved for state residents to applicants who come from other states that are participants in the program.

You should also be aware that schools that your close relatives may have attended may indeed pay some degree of attention to "legacies." How much family ties mean depends on the institution, but it is certainly worthwhile to communicate that your interest in the school was stimulated, in part, by your relative.

Yet another factor that most students must consider when applying to medical schools is cost. Yearly tuition ranges from hundreds of dollars (for state residents at some state schools) to over $26,000 (for "out-of-staters" attending the University of Colorado School of Medicine) (1). While loans are often available, you and your parents should discuss which schools on your list, if any, would be unsuitable choices due to financial constraints. The most expensive schools are not necessarily the best schools, and excluding really high-end institutions from consideration does not mean that you won't get the very finest education.

Finally, you should consider including on your applications list medical schools that offer combined degree programs of interest to you. Such programs make is possible to earn two degrees, usually in less time than it would take to earn each separately. The most common combination is the MD-PhD which typically attracts applicants with experience in, and a firm commitment to, medical research. Each year more than one hundred MD-PhD students are able to secure funding covering tuition and an added stipend through the Medical Scientist Training Program (MSTP). MD-JD (medicine-law), MD-MBA (medicine-business), and MD-MPH (medicine-public health) programs also exist. Such programs are noted in your copy of the AAMC's book on admission requirements. By applying to a large-enough number of schools, with a wide-enough range of selectivity, and with tuitions that let your dad keep the farm, you will be covering your bases fairly well. Understanding the more subtle differences between medical schools is easier after visiting. Points to consider will be discussed in Chapter 8.

GETTING THE RIGHT RECOMMENDATIONS

Recommendations from faculty members and others are an extremely important part of your application. The perspectives of the professors who presumably know you well will be taken seriously by medical school admissions committees.

Different colleges assemble final recommendations in different ways. At Brown, students were asked to request letters of recommendation from three professors or research preceptors and to submit them on standardized forms to the premedical advisor. The advisor then attached an extensive cover letter before sending the three forms to medical schools. Premedical advisors at other colleges may actually compose a composite recommendation consisting of elements of each professor's or preceptor's comments rather than sending the originals. The appropriate number of recommendations to request also varies from college to college, but usually falls between three and five. Be sure you understand how many letters you will need and the ways in which the letters may be transformed before reaching medical schools.

Regardless of whether you are asked to submit three or more recommendations, two should be from individuals able to comment on your ability and interest in science. Both recommendations may come from science course instructors, or one may be from a professor and the other from a medical researcher with whom you have worked. If your extracurricular activities do not show an obvious ability to write well, consider requesting a third recommendation from one of your liberal arts professors—perhaps one who taught creative writing or literature. You premedical advisor can guide you more carefully, of course, and should be consulted before you request any letters.

Hopefully, you will have enjoyed close relationships with faculty members during your premedical years. The best recommendations come from instructors who can comment not only on your course work, but on your special interests, your character, and your ability to relate to others. Professors from whom you have frequently sought advice in the past may be especially eager to help you with this part of your application. Even if you find that you must request a recommendation from an individual who knows you less well, make certain that you ask directly if he or she would like to write such a letter and whether this person feels he knows enough about you to do a good job. There is nothing wrong with explaining the importance of recommendations and emphasizing the limited number you can submit. It makes little sense to be evaluated by a reluctant professor, and you should look elsewhere if you get the feeling that he or she is writing solely out of obligation.

It is generally best to request letters of recommendation

from professors or from the directors of a research laboratory in which you worked. Even laboratory teaching assistants can occasionally write about an applicant with great insight, but such individuals are rare. A lower-ranking instructor should be selected only when you have enjoyed a truly unusual relationship with this person and he or she expresses a sincere desire to comment positively on your qualifications. Recommendations from relatives, friends, or community leaders outside the academic world should be avoided since these individuals are not likely to touch on some important aspects of your abilities and achievements that are relevant to your application to medical school.

THE MECHANICS OF THE APPLICATION PROCESS

Medical schools either prepare their own application forms or utilize the American Medical College Application Service (AMCAS). AMCAS, a branch of the AAMC, sends its standard application form, along with your MCAT scores, to any of the more than 90 participating schools you designate. The system allows the applicant to apply to many schools by filling out one application and, at the same time, provides medical schools with certain data about the applicant pool. Many medical schools using AMCAS will also require you to complete shorter secondary application forms at a later date. Both AMCAS and non-AMCAS applications have space for personal comments or essays. The AMCAS essay is optional, but all applicants should take advantage of the space provided to tell admissions committees more about themselves. An outstanding essay may set you apart from the crowd. Chapter 6 discusses the medical school essay in detail.

You should request applications from medical schools during March and April of your junior year. Institutions noted in *Medical School Admissions Requirements* as using the AMCAS system will accept the AMCAS application. This can be obtained by submitting an Application Request Form, available from your premedical advisor or by writing to:

AMCAS
Division of Student Services
Association of American Medical Colleges
Suite 301
1776 Massachusetts Avenue, NW
Washington, DC 20036-1989

Application forms for any non-AMCAS school can be obtained by writing directly to that school.

Although deadlines are later, plan to send out all your applications by August 1. Make sure that your college transcript or transcripts reach AMCAS before the application itself. While AMCAS will accept official transcripts beginning March 15, there is no harm in waiting until your second-semester grades can be included. In contrast, non-AMCAS schools prefer to receive a student's transcript after his or her application. Request that your college send transcripts to these schools shortly after you send the application forms. To allow you to check that transcripts have actually been sent out, ask that a copy also be mailed to your own address.

When AMCAS has received all the required information, copies of your AMCAS application will be mailed to the schools you have designated, and you will receive notification of the "transmittal date"—the date when the application was distributed.

Your MCAT scores will automatically be mailed to any AMCAS school to which you have applied. Copies for six non-AMCAS schools, which you designate when registering for the test, are included in the examination fee. Additional copies can be sent to other non-AMCAS schools by filling out another form and paying an additional fee.

If all of this sounds a bit complicated, it is. The application process is one place to allow your compulsive side some play.

Check and double-check deadlines. Keep photocopies of every form you send out. Have friends proofread your applications. Little mistakes can translate to big delays, and getting into medical school is challenging enough without having to work against your own mistakes.

The interviewing season at medical schools begins in the fall. According to AAMC figures (1), some medical schools interview as few as 10 percent of their applicants, rejecting the rest without further consideration, while other schools interview as many as 50 percent. The average is probably somewhere around 30 percent. With such a significant cut already made, those who receive interviews are part of the way toward acceptance. What happens at the interview can be quite important. Strategies for success are discussed in Chapter 7.

By convention, medical schools do not notify applicants of acceptance prior to October 15. The process continues all year. You and your classmates may receive interviews, acceptances, and rejections right up until the day medical school is slated to begin.

THE EARLY DECISION PLAN

A small percentage of applicants each year take advantage of the Early Decision Plan (EDP) and, at least initially, apply to only one medical school. The terms of the program require that you file no other applications unless you are rejected by your EDP choice. EDP applications are generally due before August 1 of junior year, and medical schools notify students of acceptance or rejection on or before October 1. If the mail brings bad news (i.e., a rejection), you are free to apply to as many other schools as you like. You can even apply for regular admission to your EDP school.

Students who take the Early Decision Plan option are generally those with an excellent chance of admission to medical school. If accepted, they avoid the expense of filing five or 10 applications and of interviewing at several schools. Best of all, they also enjoy peace of mind during senior year when most applicants are checking the mail five times a day.

The EDP is not, however, without risk. Should you be rejected, your other applications will be filed rather late in the game. At some medical schools the delay won't be a handicap, but at some schools it will. And even if you are accepted, being admitted under the EDP program means passing up the opportunity to explore other schools during interview season. My initial impressions of several schools changed significantly after I visited and spent time asking questions and seeing the cities I might be calling home for four years.

Taking full advantage of the EDP, therefore, means researching medical schools enough to be sure that your "early" choice is really your first choice. Being admitted a bit before the crowd, after all, is hardly worth passing up your chance to attend a medical school where you could have been happier.

NOTE FOR MINORITY APPLICANTS ... AND OTHERS

The percentage of minority students in medical school has not changed significantly for many years. In addition, tuitions continue to rise and threaten to make medical education an even more distant dream for those minority students who are also financially disadvantaged. As medical schools attempt to put careers in medicine within the reach of those who have traditionally had limited access, the well-prepared minority applicant will find the road to acceptance somewhat less rocky. This commitment to minority applicants recognizes that minorities are underrepresented in the medical profession and often must overcome hardships that make their achievements somewhat more impressive than numbers can show.

Black Americans, American Indians, Mexican Americans, mainland Puerto Ricans, and individuals from low-income families who gain acceptance to medical school should be aware that the rates of attrition (failure) for minorities are often higher than for the rest of the class. Whether this is because applicants have been accepted when ill-prepared or because they have not received sufficient social support once enrolled is unclear.

Minority applicants may, therefore, want to explore with medical students and administrators how minorities have fared in the classrooms and the clinics of each of the medical schools to which they apply. Your chances of success will be enhanced by your awareness of what support systems are in place for individuals with your background. Ask specifically for the rate of attrition for students in your cultural or socioeconomic group.

Minority students should also consider taking advantage of the AAMC's Medical Minority Applicant Registry (Med-MAR) which circulates information about minority students to medical schools in the United States. Individual institutions can then make further contact with students in whom they have a special interest. The Med-MAR questionnaire is filled out during the MCAT. Further information about this program and others is available by writing to:

> Minority Student Information Clearinghouse
> Association of American Medical Colleges
> Suite 200
> One Dupont Circle, NW
> Washington, DC 20036

Finally, all students should be aware that the policies that encourage minority applications to medical school are an honest attempt to provide minority students with equal access to medical education. Whether the current system is itself the fairest way to achieve that goal is the subject of continuing debate.

FINANCES

Application fees ($50 at some schools), MCAT fees, and travel-related expenses make applying to medical school quite expensive—as much as $2000. For some applicants, dealing with this financial obstacle means making a phone call home, but for many others it means a part-time job during junior year, a loan, or requests for fee waivers. Although applying to fewer schools closer to home and passing up MCAT review courses can significantly reduce the price tag, the application process is so important that students should try to find ways to finance a complete effort.

There are fee waivers available for the AMCAS application service, for applications to non-AMCAS schools, and for some MCAT review courses. Inquiries about such funding should be made directly to the organizations involved even before the application process begins. If money is going to be a problem during junior year, you should spend time as a sophomore inquiring about your options. Be sure to involve your premedical advisor who may be able to direct you to sources of funding available through your college.

Although applying to medical school will be a significant burden for some of you, it is certainly not the last, nor the greatest, financial hurdle you will confront. Financing your medical education itself is infinitely more challenging. Financial aspects of medical school are discussed in Chapter 8.

REFERENCES

1. Association of American Medical Colleges: *Medical School Admission Requirements 1985-1986*. Washington, D.C., AAMC, 1984, pp 14, 33, 101, passim.

6

The Medical School Essay

". . . you should say what you mean,"
the March Hare went on.
"I do," Alice hastily replied; "at least I mean what I say—
that's the same thing, you know."
"Not the same thing a bit!" said the Hatter (1).

LEWIS CARROLL

CHOOSING A THEME

Not every medical school will ask that you write an essay on a specific topic. Many, including schools that utilize the American Medical College Application Service (AMCAS) application form, will leave the subject up to you. Choosing an appropriate theme is important because it can shape your essay into a cohesive whole which communicates an idea rather than a list of facts or achievements.

Since there are likely to be plenty of applicants with grades and scores similar to yours, admissions committees will want to know what makes you different from the crowd. They pride themselves on the diversity of students they bring to the freshman class. Participating in high-powered medical research, achieving the black belt in karate, or playing in a jazz band all set you apart and belong in your essay.

The best essays, I believe, begin at the end—with what you have learned from your experiences. They revolve around concepts you have come to value—the physician as a person with a liberal education, the importance of individual effort in solving social problems, the role of teamwork in the fight against disease, the power of persistence. Such concepts provide a framework for discussion of the personal experiences that connect you with them. Skills you have mastered, community projects on which you have worked, places you have visited, and people with whom you have spent time all have contributed to the kind of individual you have become. Try to unify those experiences under the umbrella of greater lessons they have taught you.

Working through the experiences you feel have been most important to your development should give you a better sense of why you have chosen medicine as a career. If you followed the advice in Chapters 1, 2, and 3, you will have had practical experience to bolster your feelings about the profession. But medicine is more than emergency rooms and laboratories. If you played college football, you may have learned about leadership and teamwork. Majoring in art may have taught you a great deal about creativity and imagination. Confronting and overcoming financial obstacles may have convinced you of the power of determination. All of the understandings gained from such experiences have a place in medicine, and your essay can communicate to admissions committees that you will bring a valuable perspective to the profession.

PRESENTING YOUR STRENGTHS

The desire to explain potential weaknesses in your record too often leads to rambling essays that read like excuses. You can use the theme or themes upon which you build your essay to explain these potential problem areas and turn them into advantages. Be honest and confront, in a positive way, the issues that may concern admissions committees.

For example, an older applicant who has spent years working in industry need not write off his or her experiences as idle time. Far from it, years in marketing, sales, or research may have helped this person to solidify a commitment to closer personal contact. Experience in fields other than health care, in fact, is often directly applicable to the medical profession. Increasingly, management skills will be needed to preserve the positive aspects of medicine in the face of growing financial constraints. Those with a knowledge of law may be able to help alleviate the litigious climate in which doctors must practice "defensive medicine." Engineers may be able to apply their skills to the design of artificial organs.

Almost any problem can be seen as an experience that has taught the applicant an important lesson. The student who is applying to medical school for a second time may have learned that becoming a physician is even more important to him or her than previously imagined. This applicant may have learned something about persistence. Students with written notations of academic dishonesty on their records may understand more clearly than most the value of integrity and trust.

W. Clement Stone once said, "Every great man, every successful man, no matter what the field of endeavor, has known the magic that lies in these words: Every adversity has the seed of an equivalent or greater benefit" (2). Understanding that can make you a more successful applicant and a better physician.

THE NITTY GRITTY

The following points will help you to avoid mistakes and make full use of your application.

1. First things first. Although the AMCAS "Personal Comments" section is optional, don't leave it blank. Admissions committees may conclude that you either have nothing to say or that you are embarrassed about not being able to say it well.
2. Don't boast. There is a difference between reporting achievements of which you are rightfully proud and bragging. "As captain, I led the swim team to its best season ever," would be better put, "As captain, I was able to bring into play athletic and leadership skills which I believe helped the swim team toward an unusually successful season."
3. Limit the amount of space devoted to describing your research. The theme of the essay has to be more than a blow-by-blow discourse on your adventures in the laboratory.
4. Do not be overly critical of the health care delivery system or of health care professionals. Your well-intentioned reflections on the need for physicians more sensitive to their patients' needs may be read as the uninformed preachings of an outsider.

5. Leave out basic information found elsewhere on the application such as your date of birth or the name of your undergraduate college. Use the space provided to convey ideas rather than facts.

6. Avoid using the passive voice in your essay. Take credit for your achievements. "During my senior year *I was awarded* the Albert Lamb community service award," is less direct than stating, "During my senior year *I won* the Albert Lamb community service award.

7. The essay should look good. Single-space the text and use Liquid Paper correction fluid when correcting any mistakes. Skip two lines between paragraphs rather than indenting. Center the essay on the page and leave wide margins:

xxxxxxxxxxxxxxxxxxxxxxxxxxxxxxxxxxxxxxxxxxxxxxxxxx

xxxxxxxxxxxxxxxxxxxxxxxxxxxxxxxxxxxxxxxxxxxxxxxxxx

xxxxxxxxxxxxxxxxxxxxxxxxxxxxxxxxxxxxxxxxxxxxxxxxxx

xxxxxxxxxxxxxxxxxxxxxxxxxxxxxxxxxxxxxxxxxxxxxxxxxx

xxxxxxxxxxxxxxxxxxxxxxxxxxxxxxxxxxxxxxxxxxxxxxxxxx

xxxxxxxxxxxxxxxxxxxxxxxxxxxxxxxxxxxxxxxxxxxxxxxxxx

8. Use only the space provided and enclose no additional materials with the AMCAS application.

9. You can clarify any part of your academic record that may be confusing by drawing a line under the AMCAS essay and adding a note of explanation.

xxxxxxxxxxxxxxxxxxxxxxxxxxxxxxxxxxxxxxxxxxxxxxxxxxx

xx

xx

A note concerning my academic record:

The General Physics sequence 101 listed under advanced placement is not part of the recommended premedical sequence. For this reason, I took Physics 201, the advised course for premedical students, during my senior year. I hope this explanation prevents any confusion that the apparent duplication of General Physics might have produced.

Other application forms may allot specific spaces for this purpose.

10. Keep a photocopy of each essay you write. Other schools may ask similar questions and having the answers at hand can save you a great deal of time.
11. In addition to having your premedical advisor read and comment on your essay, recruit an English professor to proofread your work and offer suggestions. Instructors well-versed in writing can help you to polish your essay by reading for structure and grammar as well as for content.

Selected Successful Essays

The following essays were submitted by students who were accepted by more than one medical school. While each could be improved in certain ways, they all convey information not only about extracurricular activities, but about the applicant as an individual.

Essay #1 (AMCAS Personal Comments):

Sensitivity, understanding, a desire to help . . . I believe these are among the qualities which distinguish a *physician* from a technician. I can bring these qualities to the medical field.

My family life and broad-based education have given me the sensitivity that would prevent me from seeing a patient as a mere collection of symptoms. I have always been keenly aware of the feelings of those around me, and I believe such awareness would enable me to respond effectively to the needs of a patient. The ability to respond and the desire to respond are, or course, two different things, but desire to help is not an area in which I am lacking.

I think each of us has an obligation to (as Emerson put it) "leave the world a bit better whether by a healthy child, a garden patch, or a redeemed social condition." To me, this responsibility seems most appropriately carried out in the field of medicine. I am drawn to the medical profession in an instinctive sort of way as the area where I can best help others. I feel this desire to help people is a very important prerequisite to a medical career.

Up to now, I suppose the qualities I have described (sensitivity, desire to help others) might equally apply to a poet as to a physician. Like most premeds, I tend to idealize the medical profession at times, but I realize that medicine is a challenging, rigorous career. I welcome the challenge. My academic and extracurricular records show, I believe, that I can respond to a challenge. I have never shied from work in anything with which I've been involved, and most of the time I feel the challenge was met—whether it be as a fraternity Rush Captain or in getting an "A" in Chemistry 610a.

One of the more challenging aspects of the medical profession, I feel, is the need to make complex decisions under pressure. Though no decisions I have made up to now have been of the life-and-death variety, I think I have shown, particularly in my extracurricular activities, the ability to make decisions. That I was elected president of my fraternity should show that, on balance, my decisions in the rush and alumni programs and on the finance committee of that organization were judged correct by my peers.

I do not mean to ignore the scientific side of medicine. Though, as I said, a physician is more than a technician, he must be a skilled scientist in addition to being a humane, caring individual. I hope my academic record will speak adequately for my suitability as a scientist. I have taken and will continue to take a wide range of life and physical sciences, and I have managed to do well thus far. It is my further hope that my suitability for medicine is in some way reflected in my work experience. I believe I have fit in and performed well in my medically-related jobs (each of which, by the way, has strengthened my interest in medicine).

In closing, I would like to mention one other trait required of every professional, a trait which I have demonstrated (I hope not over-demonstrated) here: self-confidence.

Essay #2 (Please Write an Essay Concerning Your Extracurricular Activities and Work Experiences):

While preparing for the intellectual rigors of the medical profession through my courses at Brown, I have used my spare time as a release from structured learning. I assign a great deal of importance to my development outside as well as inside the classroom.

Freshman year, I devoted fifteen hours per week to varsity volleyball. While athletics proved an exciting way to spend my first semester at Brown, I found that the time commitment was preventing me from becoming involved in a number of other activities which I saw as more important.

Sophomore year, I began serving as a tour guide for the Bruin Club. I enjoy sharing my knowledge about Brown and my experiences there with prospective freshman. From my own experience, I realize that the impression one gets while touring a college campus is a crucial factor in determining whether he or she applies to a given school. Because I am proud of Brown and appreciative of its role in my recent growth, I feel I can present the university positively and effectively.

I have also been involved with the Student Alumni Relations Committee (SARC) for two years. This past semester, I was in charge of organizing a pilot program which matches engineering students with alumni engineers for one day externships. By allowing alumni to contribute to Brown through their experiences (rather than their pockets), the role SARC plays within the Brown community is a vital one.

Sometimes the most frustrating, but always the most rewarding, afternoon I spend is with my "little sister" Robin, a 14-year-old deaf girl with whom I communicate by sign language. By spending time with her, and by transporting other deaf children to and from the Brown campus, I have become more sensitive to the special problems the deaf community confronts. Just as Robin now functions more comfortably in the hearing world, I now find myself becoming increasingly at ease with Robin and her friends.

With whatever free time I have left, I engage in a variety of other activities. Catering for food services and tutoring physics students provides me with extra spending money. Rhythmic aerobics twice a week helps me to relax after a day of classes.

The past two summers I have worked at an overnight camp in Ontario, Canada. I found my summers as a senior counselor and an assistant unit head summers well-spent. I made many friends, formed great memories for myself, and, hopefully, provided my campers with summers of growth and fun. Working at camp taught me about dealing effectively with a wide range of people and a wide variety of problems.

Although my camping experiences are something I will always treasure, I felt this summer would be the most opportune time to spend some time with my family and get to know more about my future profession. My work at Western Pennsylvania Hospital is providing me with greater insight into the everyday life and responsibilities of physicians. I currently serve as a research assistant in the Burn Unit, but have also been observing surgery on a daily basis. Through such experiences, and by accompanying physicians on rounds, I have begun to obtain a more complete picture of my chosen profession. Together with my volunteer work at Rhode Island Hospital, my employment at West Penn has made me more educated about many aspects of medical training and practice.

Essay #3 (Type or Attach a Typed Statement Setting Forth Any Information About Yourself Which Would Be of Interest to the Committee on Admission):

My life experiences have convinced me that I wish to devote my professional life to the pursuit of the scientific method in service to humanity. Medicine appeals to me as a profession because it involves personal contact and utilizes scientific methodology and technology. Whether medicine will lead to clinical work, research, or a combination of both, I seek the gratification of a profession that involves helping people and working with colleagues.

As a biochemistry major at the University of Pennsylvania, I developed scientific knowledge and the ability to think as a scientist. A major use to which I put scientific knowledge has been in research. One of my most significant accomplishments has been screening a human DNA library for a family of actin genes, working at the Laboratory of Molecular Carcinogenesis of the National Cancer Institute (NCI). I successfully cloned at least five distinct DNA fragments, thus opening the door for further research into the genetics of actin. The report on the characterization of one of the clones, entitled "A Human Beta-Actin Pseudogene Lacks Intervening Sequences: A Processed Gene," has been submitted for publication. Last summer, at the Immunology Branch of the NCI, my work involved studying the evolution of major histocompatibility complex (MHC) genes by Southern blotting wild mice genomic DNA using specific Class I and Class II MHC cDNA fragments as hybridization probes. This year, as part of my curriculum, I will be working at the Department of Pathology of the University of Pennsylvania School of Medicine studying gene expression and regulation. My project involves constructing and screening a genomic library from afibrinogenemic patients, who produce no fibrinogen but have the three fibrinogen genes without major structural rearrangements. What appeals to me about science and research is the way in which one can answer questions using procedures that are clever but relatively simple once mastered. In addition to research, I have had the opportunity at the National Institutes of Health to see surgery and to attend seminars on disease. These experiences confirm my desire to pursue a medical career that involves patients and may involve research.

My Penn experience has been not only scientific but has also broadened my view of man and society. Through the study of the humanities and the social sciences, and in my extracurricular activities, I have derived other kinds of satisfaction which also involve seeking knowledge and applying it to new situations. My activities have also provided contact and interaction with people and have given me opportunities to assume leadership. As a freshman, I wrote a socio-political column for the *Penn Press*, a Penn student publication, based on investigations I did into socialist movements and religious cults. The column reached the student community and provided an open forum for my views. A major extracurricular activity has been the founding and operation of Musical Productions, a musical management and booking agency. The agency's success resulted from my ability to represent talented musicians and promote them in an appealing manner. My motivation was not only financial, but also brought the reward of seeing the product of my initiative. I have brought unknown musical groups recognition in nightclubs in Philadelphia and other cities, and some have gone on to cut records. In addition, my organization gave me unique opportunities to serve the community. For instance, I provided entertainment for charity dance marathons and benefit concerts.

School, research, and extracurricular activities have required a great deal of responsibility; however, I have not let them preclude other important aspects of my life. I maintain close relationships with many friends and find time for reading, athletics, and recreation. I feel that all my activities have helped me grow as a person, have been rewarding, and have given me confidence in my abilities. I look forward to moving on and devoting my energies to the field of medicine in which I can help others and find fulfillment.

Essay #4 (Type or Attach a Typed Statement Setting Forth Any Information About Yourself Which Would Be of Interest to the Committee on Admission):

A person would not normally begin an essay such as this by stating his or her height, but the fact that I am 6'-10" has had an enormous effect on my life. It has structured my life more than any other personal characteristic. Its effects range from my relations with others to the sports in which I participate.

First I would like to explain how I feel my height affects my relations with others. I do not think of myself as a freak of nature. First of all, I am not that tall. Secondly, I am a motivated, confident individual who is not self-conscious about his height. I do realize, however, that others are not completely at ease with a person my size. Yet my attitude towards my height as well as my general nature are such that this has never amounted to much of a problem.

The athletic restrictions of my height are more obvious. While I enjoy many sports, basketball seemed like the most logical route to follow. Basketball, I love, not only as a sport but also for the opportunities which it has offered to me. I have travelled fairly extensively and have met a wide variety of people. Playing for a college team has taught me several things. Anyone who has been a premed major playing a major intercollegiate sport understands well the time compromise one must sacrifice between lab time, practice time, study time, and days on the road. I can honestly say that during the basketball season, which runs from the middle of October on into March, I consistently put in a 14- to 16-hour work day. This experience has not only taught me to budget my time but it has enabled me to prove to myself that I can work successfully under extreme pressure. In fact I actually enjoy the pressure, as well as the feeling of accomplishment. Secondly, a college basketball team consists of ten to twenty men who spend the greater part of six months together. The typical team contains a variety of personalities and mixed emotions. Learning to relate to people becomes essential, not only for the good of the team, but to preserve one's sanity.

Before closing I would like to stress that I have been determined not to let my athletics interfere with either my academics or my desire to become a doctor. As I stated in the previous questions, I have worked in two hospitals, viewed surgery in a third, and have done independent research on total knee replacements. One of the hospital jobs was work as an intern in the emergency room at the Lowrance Hospital in Mooresville, N.C. My function was to observe and help with various procedures, such as checking blood pressures and running EKGs. The other hospital job was at the Miller Orthopaedic Clinic in

Charlotte, N.C. Here I was able to observe and talk with many patients suffering from a wide variety of bone related problems. Most of the doctors specialized, and I was allowed to work with a different one each day. Scholastically, I have received several honors including the ODK and AED honorary societies and have always maintained a goal to excel in both academics and athletics. In this regard being chosen third team Academic All-American was most satisfying. My long term goal, however, is to become a doctor. As in anything worthwhile, medicine requires a great deal of work, yet it is a career choice which I feel both excited about and suited for.

Essay #5 (Type or Attach a Typed Statement Setting Forth Any Information About Yourself Which Would Be of Interest to the Committee on Admission):

Although college has afforded me the opportunity to explore and contemplate various careers, I have carefully decided to pursue a career as a physician. Medicine attracts me because it has the potential to combine my interests in basic science and medicine with my desire to work with people. My initial interest in medicine occurred during my high school years, and has been strengthened over the past two years as a result of various clinical and research experiences.

While I worked as a volunteer in the Emergency Ward of Massachusetts General Hospital, I had the opportunity to interact with patients who were nervous or perhaps unable to speak English, besides being ill. Working in a psychiatric hospital as a counselor's aide allowed me to explore an area of medicine that I had had little experience in clinically or academically. I found psychiatry to be a very challenging area of medicine, as I realized that it is often more difficult to heal the mind than physical wounds. Both of these experiences helped to reinforce my belief that a trusting relationship between physician and patient plays an important role in the subsequent progress of the patient's mental and physical health. Feeling that these clinical experiences were valuable, I decided to explore other areas of interest to help me better define my career goals.

A career which combined health and medicine with government was also another possibility that I was considering. Wishing to explore this option, I decided to take a temporary leave from my part time job at the psychiatric hospital to serve as a research assistant for the Science Resource Office of the Massachusetts State Legislature. During this internship, I prepared a report which concerned child abuse programs and centers in Massachusetts. Although the work I was doing was worthwhile and interesting, it did not allow me to directly interact with the people that my work was benefiting.

Although my interests in the biomedical sciences were very strong, I also had an attraction towards the field of chemistry. I felt that since I enjoyed this subject, that my undergraduate years were the best time for me to pursue it. Owing to this additional interest I decided to undertake a research project in organic chemistry. My project involved the synthesis and structural analysis of a group of compounds, beta-keto acids, which are intermediates in fatty acid metabolism. I will continue my chemistry major at Wellesley College by accepting the Chemistry Department's invitation to do honors work in physical chemistry. Using nuclear magnetic resonance spectroscopy, I will study the structure of dinucleotide molecules in the presence of metal ions.

Since I derive satisfaction from research, I am considering a combined career in medicine and clinical research. In an effort to explore and gain experience in clinical research, I decided to pursue a research project in an area of medical science. This summer I am working with an immunopathologist on a project which is attempting to explain a correlation between prostaglandin levels and the suppression of an autoimmune disease, systemic lupus erythematosus (SLE). At this time, I am not ready to decide if I wish to pursue a combined career in medicine and clinical research, but regardless of my decision I am anxious to begin the study of medicine. My main priority is to pursue a career as a physician, with the hope that my experiences this summer, and during my first year in medical school will aid me in making the correct decision concerning a combined career in medicine and clinical research.

REFERENCES

1. Carroll L: *Alice's Adventures in Wonderland and Through the Looking Glass.* Middlesex, England, Puffin Books, 1982, p 94.
2. As quoted in Allen RG: *Creating Wealth.* New York, Simon & Schuster, 1986, p 291.

7

The Interview

"I have often thought that the best way to define a man's character would be to seek out the particular mental or moral attitude in which, when it came upon him, he felt himself most deeply and intensely active and alive. At such moments there is a voice inside which speaks and says: 'This is the real me!'"(1).

WILLIAM JAMES

HOW FAR HAVE I COME?

As discussed in Chapter 5, medical schools vary in the percentage of applicants to whom they offer interviews. The average is approximately 30 percent (2); thus, the student who makes it to this final stage of the application process is already part of a select group. His or her basic academic record has passed the test. Although some medical schools have seats for only five percent of those who apply, they must often offer admission to a higher percentage to compensate for those students who will decide to enroll elsewhere. As many as half of those interviewed, therefore, may be offered admission.

For some applicants, the interview will serve mainly to assure the admission committee that no glaring weakness in the applicant's character or interpersonal skills has been missed. For others, however, the interview is an opportunity to strengthen their candidacies by demonstrating poise, character, enthusiasm, and self-confidence. In every case, the interview has the potential of significantly influencing the committee's final decision, and no one should take it lightly.

THE RIGHT MINDSET

Whenever my father detected any apprehension in my voice as I prepared for a first date, he always advised, "Be yourself." Presumably, this meant allowing my strengths and weaknesses to flow freely during the evening. All I had to do was "be myself." My father theorized that, with all the facts on the table, only meaningful relationships would develop. The concept was attractive because it required no preparation—I was already myself, I didn't have to work at it.

I stopped believing in my dad's theory because I found that second dates were hard to come by. The problem with "being yourself" is that it asks too much of the listener. It presumes that he or she is sensitive, has insight, and is willing to think in-depth about what is being said. That's asking a lot of a cheerleader on a first date.

Medical school interviews may, in some ways, be like first dates. The interviewers are faced with a series of 10- to 60-minute encounters with highly motivated and talented young men and women. Your interviewer may not have the time, even if he or she has a desire, to seek out explanations for weaknesses in the way you present yourself. With a large applicant pool still left to choose from, relatively small mistakes can be enough to make an interviewer less excited about your candidacy. Your key to success is being well-prepared for the interview so that you present your strengths with confidence and charm. "Being yourself" is fine on the college green, but your medical school interview requires that you be your best.

SCHEDULING

Scheduling your time properly can make your interviewing season a more sane period for you. If you are invited to interview at a number of schools in the same area, you may be able to arrange a convenient series of days to travel to that part of the country. The high cost associated with interviewing in cities far from home makes it advisable to combine several interviews into one trip. Most schools have fairly flexible schedules allowing you to pick from several days on which to visit.

Although it is generally considered proper form to wait until a medical school contacts you, it is possible to request an interview and tour if you have scheduled a visit to another school in the area. Such requests should be made in writing to the Dean of Admissions and should indicate the dates you will be available.

Some medical schools offer the option of a regional interview by an alumnus close to your home. Although taking advantage of this opportunity may be attractive because of financial factors, remember that actually visiting medical schools will give you much more information about their locations, facilities, and students.

Students who are lucky enough to be accepted by a medical school early in the season generally cancel their trips to schools they are no longer considering. However, if financial concerns are not great or if the schools are nearby, keeping your appointments will provide additional interview practice. In fact, you may be pleasantly surprised by the atmosphere at a school you had ranked low on your list and may even change your mind about which school to attend.

Once interview appointments have been arranged, any necessary changes should be made well in advance of the scheduled days. You should explain the reason for your request to be interviewed at another time. Always be patient and courteous when talking with staff members on the phone. If circumstances delay you on the day of your interview, telephone ahead and explain why you will be late. When possible, plan to arrive a few hours before your appointment. The extra time will give you a chance to get oriented and to relax.

PREPARATION

Getting there is the smaller part of your responsibility. Getting ready is the bulk of it. There are a number of steps you should take to prepare for each interview. First, you should be familiar enough with your academic record and, if applicable, your medical research to field questions about either with ease. Review your transcript, making sure you remember the topics that were covered by each course. Be certain you understand and can explain the principles upon which your research was based.

In addition to reviewing your record and your research, you should try to arrange mock interviews with your premedical advisor or with other professors. These mock interviews, if well done, can help make you more at ease with the tone of a typical medical school interview. Most premedical advisors know the most frequently asked questions and can get you thinking about the answers. You should feel comfortable fielding questions such as:

Why do you want to study medicine?

Why choose medicine over some other career in health? Dentistry? Public health? Nursing?

What field of medicine interests you most?

What will you do if you fail to gain admission to medical school this year? Will you reapply? How would you spend the interim year?

How do you spend your time outside the classroom?

Would you tell me about your family?

How do you plan to fit a husband (or wife) and children in with your career?

Are you aware of the level of difficulty of medical school? Are you sure you can handle that kind of pressure?

What are your thoughts on euthanasia? On abortion?

What are the greatest problems facing American medicine?

What other medical schools have you applied to? Have you been accepted anywhere? Where would you most like to go?

Why is this medical school of interest to you?

What do you see yourself doing in five years? In ten or 15?

How do you plan to finance your medical education?

Explain your medical research to me. Did you enjoy it?

Would you like research to be part of your career?

You should also consult students already accepted at, or attending, various medical schools. Different schools tend to have different structures in place for the day applicants spend interviewing, and those who have gone through the process should be able to let you know what to expect. Some colleges, in fact, have files of interview descriptions which have been filled out by students on their return to campus. Inquire about such a resource with your premedical advisor and with advisors at other nearby schools. Knowing the routine at a given institution can make you more relaxed and can give you clues as to whether any special preparation might be in order.

Finally, since your interviewer will almost certainly ask whether you have any questions he or she might be able to answer, you should prepare several questions that demonstrate your interest in that school. You can use each school's catalogue or bulletin to identify departments, programs, or parts of the curriculum that are of particular interest to you and are not thoroughly explained.

WHAT TO SAY AND WHAT NOT TO SAY

Conveying enthusiasm about a career in medicine and expressing pride in your past accomplishments will go a long way toward establishing a good rapport with your interviewer. Try to relax and interact with him or her as a person.

You should be particularly careful not to compromise your honesty in any way. Do not be afraid to paint an accurate picture of your level of knowledge and avoid exaggerating your participation in extracurricular events. Doctors are particularly sensitive to maintaining the integrity of the medical profession, and any hint that you would violate a trust can seriously damage your chances for admission.

Be willing to acknowledge that you still have a great deal of learning to do. No one expects that you will have achieved a command of anatomy or that you will have made a firm commitment to a specialty area of medical practice. "I don't know" and "I'm not sure yet" are valid responses to questions for which you do not have sufficient information.

While it is important to be candid, some things are better addressed in other settings. If you are discontented with your undergraduate school, if you find yourself interviewing at Research Medical School and hated your research, or if you're still wrestling with whether your parents provided 51 percent of your motivation to be a doctor, work it out in a bar with good friends.

Knowing what not to say includes knowing when not to say it. Some medical schools have portions of the interview disguised as casual interactions. These can include lunches or tours. At no time should you be flip, sarcastic, or grouchy. One well-known institution stations medical students outside the admissions office to answer questions and to relate their impressions of applicants to the admissions committee. Don't be paranoid, but don't be careless.

ATTIRE

Dress conservatively. A man should wear a suit or blazer and slacks, always with a tie. Loafers or dress shoes are fine;

clogs, sandals, or sneakers are not acceptable. A woman should wear a suit, skirt, or dress and tone down her makeup and jewelry. Designer labels should be where they belong—inside clothing. The key is to avoid offending anyone with your taste, and conservative garb is always in style around medical institutions.

Ask your premedical advisor to preview the exact clothing and jewelry you will be wearing to your interviews. Trendy items are sometimes difficult to recognize when you're participating in the trend. An impartial assessment of your "interview outfit" can help you to avoid mistakes. Little things may make a difference, and you've come too far to let them get in the way.

AFTER THE INTERVIEW

Although, it's not at all clear that it helps, remembering your interviewer's name and sending him or her a thank you note for the time he spent talking with you can't hurt. The "thank you" might read as follows:

Dear Dr. Jones,

Thank you for the time you spent with me discussing my application to Tufts University School of Medicine. I enjoyed touring the school and speaking with students, and I was able to get answers to many of my questions.

I look forward to hearing from the Admissions Committee.

Sincerely,

Robert Applicant

After completing your interviews, you will have done as much as possible to gain admission to medical school. The wait for final decisions on your applications can be very stressful, but, as hard as the next weeks and months might be, you should catch your breath and try to relax. You've done your job to the best of your ability, and now the admissions committees will do the rest of the work.

REFERENCES

1. Bartlett J: *Bartlett's Familiar Quotations*. Boston, Little, Brown and Company, 1968, p 792 as quoted from *The Letters of William James*, vol. 1, p 199.
2. Association of American Medical Colleges: *Medical School Admission Requirements 1985-1986*. Washington, D.C., AAMC, 1984, passim.

8

Once You Make It

"Success is not something that can be measured or worn on a watch or hung on the wall. It is not the esteem of colleagues, or the admiration of the community, or the appreciation of patients. Success is the certain knowledge that you have become yourself, the person you were meant to be from all time. That should be reward enough" (1).

DR. GEORGE SHEEHAN

MAKING A FINAL DECISION

Although some of the successful applicants to medical school each year receive a single acceptance, others are courted by a number of institutions. Choosing a medical school from among several to which you have been accepted is one of the more pleasant tasks in the admissions process. Some of the criteria upon which to base that selection, such as yearly tuition and the opportunity to enroll in a combined degree program, were discussed in Chapter 5. The varying amounts of financial aid available may also influence your choice. But medical schools differ in other ways, and each school's special characteristics can impact on your contentment as a student and your development as a professional.

One of these is the school's reputation. While you may or may not be swayed by a school's perceived rank among the nation's 117 medical schools, you should be aware that becoming associated with a particularly well-respected institution does offer certain advantages. Such a school is likely to attract top students and faculty members and may provide an unusually stimulating environment in which to learn. Since medical professionals are not immune to the influence of reputation, students from Yale, Harvard, Columbia, and the like might find summer positions in research laboratories and hospitals easier to come by. The best residency programs may be within closer reach.

Different medical schools also emphasize different aspects of the profession. Some highlight the importance of medical research and strive to interest students in careers in academic medicine. Others stress primary care of patients and tend to produce unusual numbers of family practitioners. If you are like most students, you have not decided the exact path your career will take. Still, should your interests seem best served by the resources and role models at one of the medical schools to which you have been accepted, you may be most comfortable studying at that school.

As important as reputation and research or primary care emphasis can be, your choice of a medical school should also take into account the environment in which you will be expected to study. If you interviewed at a number of medical schools, you may have noted that students at certain institutions seem to be under greater academic pressure than at others. The number of scheduled classroom hours, the placement of exams in the school calendar, and the frequency of overnight call during clinical rotations all contribute to the level of intensity at a given school.

How prominently grading policies figure in the pressure formula is debatable. Many medical schools have adopted Pass/Fail or Honors/Pass/Fail grading systems, but others have continued to evaluate students with traditional letter grades. While letter grades may seem like unnecessary stressors, some educators report that residency program directors ultimately insist on letter-grade equivalents of whatever form of grading appears on a student's transcript. Using traditional grading, they argue, allows students to evaluate their academic standing accurately and places good students at a competitive advantage when seeking residency positions.

The grading policy and academic schedule, along with other important characteristics of each medical school in the United States, have been compiled by the American Association of Medical Colleges in its *AAMC Curriculum Directory*. The book is available for a fee (currently $7.50 shipped book rate) by writing to:

> Association of American Medical Colleges
> Attn: Membership and Publication Orders
> One Dupont Circle, NW, Suite 200
> Washington, D.C. 20036

Appreciating the levels of stress medical students face at the schools to which you have been admitted is only half the battle. Once you know where the high pressure environments are, you will need to decide whether you wish to avoid them. People react differently to stress, and it may or may not be to your advantage to enroll in a school where student life is more relaxed.

In addition to the level of academic pressure, the medical school atmosphere can be influenced by the school's physical setting. Certain medical schools benefit from being situated on the same campus as an undergraduate school, a school of law, or a school of business. The opportunity to interact with students who are studying other disciplines can make whatever free time is available more enjoyable. Studying in a favorite city or close to your hometown can make days off especially pleasant.

Even after assessing the factors discussed above, you may wish to schedule a longer visit to the schools you are giving the most serious consideration. Sitting through a day or two of classes, talking with students in their dorm rooms, and exploring the city can go a long way toward helping you select the medical school that is best for you.

A NOTE ON HOUSING

Medical schools generally offer students housing close by. While financial considerations may make university housing the only alternative, students who have the resources to consider other alternatives should weigh the advantages and disadvantages of dormitory life.

One of the benefits of living in a medical school dormitory is that it makes getting to know your classmates easier. There is a certain camaraderie, which comes from late-night study breaks and midnight pizza runs, that is difficult to capture between classes during the school day. Living with your classmates also means that you can wander across the suite and borrow notes from yesterday's lecture. Last-minute cramming sessions are just down the hall.

The proximity of university housing to the library and to classes can also be an advantage. Being able to roll out of bed 15 minutes before biochemistry class can make fighting 30 minutes of traffic to commute to school look like a very weak option.

Still, there is a downside to dormitory life. Living at a medical school makes it difficult to escape the constant pressure of student life. One of the advantages my housemates and I most appreciated when we moved from the Hopkins dorm to a suburban townhouse was the sense it allowed us of going home after the school day. Our bedrooms looked out on wooded land instead of the hospital dome, and our apartment became a safe haven from the pathology lab and the lecture hall.

Living away from Johns Hopkins also placed us among people who had nothing to do with medicine. Bunking with visiting physicians, public health graduate students, and two hundred medical students had become a bit oppressive. It was refreshing to see children racing tricycles after a day spent looking at stacks of histology slides. Talking with neighbors about politics and business made us feel human.

Whatever the advantages and disadvantages we saw to living in on-campus versus off-campus housing, we all agreed that living as a group was important. Communal suffering is more tolerable than suffering alone, and being able to curse our workload while throwing a Nerf football around the house made the next two hours of study time more bearable.

Finally, before deciding where to live, be sure either to tour the available school housing or speak with students living there. The condition of the building may make it a less attractive alternative.

FINANCES

AAMC figures show that first-year medical students (attending school out of state) spent an average of $14,060 for tuition and all other expenses during the 1983-1984 academic year (2). For some students, full financial support from parents makes seeking other sources of funding unnecessary. But for the majority, making medical education feasible means securing scholarships or loans.

Scholarships are gifts—cash awards or tuition waivers that need not be repaid. The first place to look for such funding is at the financial aid office of each medical school to which you have been accepted. Medical schools rarely, however, offer scholarships that cover a student's total financial need. A cash award or tuition waiver is almost always available only as part of a total financial aid package including loans that must be repaid.

Students with extreme financial difficulties (zero resources) may qualify for the Scholarship Program for First-Year Students of Exceptional Financial Need. Under this program, a small number of first-year students are granted full tuition and expense money for one year. Although these scholarships are federally funded, they are dispensed through medical schools, and application should be made through the financial aid officer at the school you plan to attend.

Minority students can apply for National Medical Fellowships available to black Americans, American Indians, Mexican Americans, and mainland Puerto Ricans. Limited awards are generally given to first- and second-year students on the basis of financial need. Send requests to:

Scholarship Program
National Medical Fellowships, Inc.
Room 1820
250 West 57th Street
New York, NY 10107

Far more common than scholarships are government-backed loans including Guaranteed Student Loans (GSL), Health Education Assistance Loans (HEAL), Health Professions Student Loans (HPSL), National Direct Student Loans (NDSL), and Parental Loans to Undergraduate Students (PLUS). Although these loans are each sponsored by the government, the terms of each, including rates of interest, differ greatly. Being an intelligent consumer of loan money requires a familiarity with the subtleties of each loan program.

GSL: Guaranteed Student Loans are awarded on the basis of financial need. Interest (currently eight percent) does not accrue until after your graduation from medical school, and you may defer beginning to repay the loan for two years during your residency. The maximum loan is $5,000 per year and $25,000 in total.

HEAL: Health Education Assistance Loans are regarded by some financial aid officers as "expensive" money. Although you may defer beginning to repay the loan until after your residency, interest begins to accrue immediately when the loan is taken. The rate of interest varies quarterly as the 91-day Treasury bill rate plus 3.5 percent. The maximum loan is $20,000 per year and $80,000 in total.

HPSL: Health Professions Student Loans are awarded to students with exceptional financial need. You may defer repayment until after your residency training. Interest (currently nine percent) does not accrue until you begin paying back the loan. The maximum loan is tuition plus $2500 per year. There is no specified limit on the total support available from this source.

NDSL: National Direct Student Loans are awarded on the basis of financial need. Like Guaranteed Student Loans, interest (currently five percent) does not accrue until after your graduation, and you can delay beginning to repay the loan for two years of residency training. The maximum total funding available is $12,000.

PLUS: Parental Loans to Undergraduate Students are also labelled by some as "expensive" money. Interest begins to accrue immediately when the loan is taken. PLUS funding is less risky than is HEAL funding since the loans carry a guaranteed rate of interest (currently 12 percent). You may defer beginning to pay the principal, but not the interest on the loan, until after your residency. The maximum loan is $3,000 per year and $15,000 in total.

Another way to finance medical education is by promising future service in exchange for tuition and other expenses. The United States Public Health Service provides funding to a limited number of medical students who, following training, must later serve in communities whose population is without adequate medical care. Interested students should obtain further information from:

National Health Service Corps
    Scholarship Program
Bureau of Health Care Delivery and Assistance
Room 7-16, Parklawn Building
5600 Fishers Lane
Rockville, MD 20857

The various branches of the armed forces also offer funding for service. Tuition and expenses, plus an annual stipend, are provided in return for future years of active duty. Complete information on the programs can be obtained from the appropriate service branch at one of the following addresses:

Navy Recruiting Command
4015 Wilson Boulevard
Arlington, VA 22203

Department of the Army
Attn: SGPE-PDM-S
1900 Half Street, SW
Washington, D.C. 20324

Headquarters, USAF Recruiting Service
Directorate of Health Professions Recruiting
Randolph AFB, TX 78150

In addition to the financial aid offered by medical schools and the government, scholarships or loans are often available to individuals from a given city or town, to members of various organizations or fraternities, to handicapped students, and to those affiliated with a particular religion. Medical school financial aid officers and your premedical advisor may be able to put you in touch with such sources of support.

Students from your hometown or your college who are already attending medical school should also be consulted. They will sometimes be aware of additional sources of funding.

REFERENCES

1. As quoted in Allen RG: *Creating Wealth*. New York, Simon & Schuster, 1986, p 294.
2. Association of American Medical Colleges: *Medical School Admission Requirements 1985-1986*. Washington, D.C., AAMC, 1984, p 42.

9

If You Don't
Make It

*"Someday I hope to enjoy enough of what the world calls
success so that someone will ask me, 'What's the secret of it?'
I shall say simply this: 'I get up when I fall down'"* (1).

PAUL HARVEY

THE ADMISSIONS COMMITTEE REGRETS TO INFORM YOU...

After investing so many years in becoming a physician, finding the door to American medical education closed stimulates a variety of emotions. You may be angry that admissions committees could so coolly pass judgment on your future. You may be jealous of colleagues who gain acceptance to multiple medical schools. If you sense that you devoted too little time to your premedical studies or to the application process, you may regret your lack of discipline.

One of the most common emotions felt by rejected applicants is anxiety. As discussed in Chapter 3, the premedical curriculum prepares students specifically for medical school. Many students have not considered other career options, especially if their academic records seemed to promise medical school admission. Having to reassess whether their goals are within reach can be very stressful.

As difficult as it is to remain composed when career plans are frustrated, it is important to look rationally at the factors that might be behind your rejection. Rejection letters should not be taken as commentaries on your character or your commitment. Many unsuccessful applicants are highly motivated and are capable of completing medical school and becoming caring, competent physicians. What rejection letters do mean is that some elements of your background—academic and otherwise—did not make a positive enough impression on admissions committees. Identifying those elements will allow you to put your rejection in perspective and to make plans for the future.

WHAT WENT WRONG?

The intricacies of the medical school admissions process make it difficult to know with certainty the reasons for your

109

rejection. Since all medical schools take notice of certain elements of a candidate's application, however, reviewing these parts of your academic performance and extracurricular activities can disclose weaknesses. In addition, critically evaluating your performance during various phases of the admissions process itself can uncover other deficiencies that may have impacted on your chances.

Make use of all the resources available to you as you analyze why you did not meet with greater success. You should seek your premedical advisor's opinion about which aspects of your candidacy were likely to have been the trouble areas. Medical school administrators may also be willing to discuss your applications with you. Contact each school to which you applied and ask to speak with the Director of Admissions.

One potential problem area is grades and MCAT scores. Although you should already have a sense of where these objective measures place you on the ladder of applicants to medical school, being rejected from several schools requires that you reassess how much of a deficit your academic credentials may have been. For example, your belief that borderline MCAT scores would be forgiven because of your high grade point average may have been erroneous.

It is possible that your chances for admission were lessened by failure to demonstrate a commitment to the medical profession. An applicant who spends no time working in a hospital or participating in medical research may find it difficult to convince admissions committees that his or her decision to become a physician is well-grounded.

While your academic record and extracurricular activities are important components of your application, your success as a candidate for admission also depends on your performance during the admissions process itself.

You must decide whether you applied to a sufficient number of schools and whether you chose the correct range of schools. If your grades or scores are average and you sought admission to only five medical schools or to only highly selective medical schools, it may be that applying to a larger number or a wider range of medical schools would have brought greater success.

The medical school essay also carries weight with admissions committees. An unorthodox, controversial, or very poorly written personal statement may have tipped the scales of admission against your acceptance. Ask your premedical advisor as well as advisors at colleges nearby to offer their comments on what you wrote.

If you were interviewed by one or more medical schools, you should question whether you were particularly ill-prepared or ill-at-ease during your interactions with medical school representatives. As discussed in Chapter 7, students making it to this final stage of the application process are part of a select group. Being rejected after a personal interview does not necessarily mean that you made a poor impression on your interviewer, but the possibility must be considered.

Finally, applications that are received late may be reviewed by admissions committees at a time in the admissions season when most of the seats in the first year class are filled. If your applications were submitted just under the wire, you lost the competitive advantage enjoyed by students who completed their applications during the summer or early fall.

Recognizing some of the potential weaknesses in your application can help you in two ways. First, by understanding better the possible reasons you did not meet with success, you can avoid seeing your rejection as a commentary on your character. Second, by identifying problem areas, you will be able to design a plan to make your admission to medical school more likely should you choose to reapply.

WHAT NOW?

An unsuccessful attempt to gain admission to medical school means that the price tag—in time, effort, and dollars—associated with medical education is now higher. What to do next depends on how important becoming a physician is to you.

The difficulty that you may confront when assessing the depth of your motivation to attend medical school is that opting not to try again can feel like surrendering. Even if you selected the medical profession half-heartedly, entering another field after being rejected from medical school may tug at your pride.

There is no easy way to step back from a goal that has been with you for years. Deciding how much more energy you are willing to expend toward that goal, however, is no job for your ego. It requires a rational evaluation of the level of your commitment to medicine and the degree of interest you may have in other careers.

After careful consideration of your motivations and goals, you may decide that pursuing a medical career even more vigorously, and again without any promise of success, involves more than you are willing to invest. Students who reapply to medical school in the United States generally spend at least one year bolstering their credentials. Attending a foreign medical school may require learning a second language and studying medicine for as long as seven years, all without a guaranteed opportunity to practice medicine in this country.

Students who are unwilling to make such a large investment should consider other career options that provide some of the same satisfactions enjoyed by physicians. Becoming an optometrist, physician's assistant, physical therapist, clinical psychologist, or lawyer offers close contact with people. A career spent as a PhD working on medical or basic science research brings into play the ability to understand and interpret scientific principles. Being trained as a hospital administrator or a pharmacist provides access to the hospital environment.

If, after considering the alternatives to medical education, you remain committed to becoming a physician, there are ways to pursue your career goal. Each year thousands of would-be physicians apply to American medical schools for a second, third, or fourth time. Others apply to medical schools in foreign countries.

REAPPLYING TO AMERICAN MEDICAL SCHOOLS

While gaining admission to medical school is less likely as a reapplicant than as a first-time applicant, statistics from the Association of American Medical Colleges show that a substantial number of individuals previously rejected by medical schools ultimately gain admission. Those reapplying during the year immediately following their first attempt fare best, but even applicants rejected three times in the past sometimes meet with success. The following data for 1984 give some indication of the odds you face (Personal communication, AAMC staff member, March 1986):

All applicants	47.8% accepted
Second-time applicants who first applied in 1983	39% accepted
Second-time applicants who first applied before 1983	28.9% accepted
Third- or fourth-time applicants	32.6% accepted

Beating the reapplication odds demands a great deal more than submitting your applications for a second look. Few students who fail to strengthen their candidacies meet with success as second-time applicants. You should plan to spend time in the year you are reapplying to medical school correcting the deficiencies you and your premedical advisor identify in your credentials.

You may decide, for example, to retake the MCAT (after extensive preparation) or to repeat key science courses in which your performance was less than impressive. Excelling in additional upper-level coursework at a nearby college might demonstrate more clearly your ability to handle especially challenging material. Some students take full-time positions working in hospitals or research laboratories in order to highlight their commitment to the medical profession and to provide a stronger foundation for their decisions to become physicians.

It is also possible to begin pursuing a graduate degree in the sciences or in public health during the year following your rejection. However, medical school admission is far from guaranteed during or after completion of the degree program, and such extended study should only be undertaken if you would be content to finish the course of study and make use of the background it provides.

In addition to bolstering your credentials for admission to medical school, you should also pay particularly close attention to putting in a strong performance during the admissions process itself. Plan to complete your applications by summer's end. If you previously applied to too few medical schools, or only those that are very selective, take additional care to select a larger number or wider range of schools. Your premedical advisor should be willing to help you with a careful review of your revised medical school essay and to suggest ways you can tune up your interviewing skills.

Even while you are reapplying to American medical schools, you should be exploring the last-resort option of foreign medical study. Should you fail for a second time to gain medical school admission in the United States, you will be able to more intelligently make the decision whether to matriculate as a medical student in another country.

FOREIGN MEDICAL STUDY

Studying medicine outside the United States is a risky venture. Many American medical educators feel that the quality of instruction at the foreign medical schools most popular with American students is inadequate, and there is no guarantee that you will be permitted to return to this country as a practicing physician. These uncertainties make it essential for you to investigate the implications of matriculating outside the United States.

The requirements for admission to foreign medical schools vary widely. Some schools require only the documented completion of premedical studies, while others also evaluate applicants by means of special entrance examinations. It is often necessary for applicants to demonstrate proficiency in the language in which lectures will be given.

Figures from the Association of American Medical Colleges (AAMC) indicate that a large percentage of Americans who attend foreign medical schools enroll in either St. George's University (Grenada), Universidad Autonoma de Guadalajara (Mexico), or Universidad del Noreste (Mexico) (2).

The specific conditions of admission, as well as curricula, of these and many other foreign medical schools are catalogued in the *World Directory of Medical Schools* published by the World Health Organization (WHO) (3). The directory also lists the name of the medical degree each school awards and the traditional training and licensure procedures which follow graduation. Only students who attend medical schools listed in the WHO directory are eligible for later transfer into an American medical school or to practice medicine in this country. Every student considering studying outside the United States should order the directory (currently $19.00, including postage) by writing to:

> United Nations Bookshop
> The United Nations
> Room G.A. 32B
> New York, NY 10017

A number of placement agencies, charging hundreds or thousands of dollars to find clients seats in foreign medical school classes, currently advertise their services in newspapers and magazines. Very few, if any, of these agencies hold special sway with foreign medical schools, and you can probably achieve the same results by writing letters of interest to the foreign consulates of the schools you are considering.

Getting into a foreign medical school is the easy part. Attending a foreign medical school is harder. Faculties and facilities are sometimes inadequate and make learning difficult (2). Students must also adjust to the language and customs of a different country. Far away from home, some feel isolated and alone. The lack of any assurance that an American graduate from a foreign medical school (a foreign medical graduate, or FMG) will have the opportunity to practice medicine in the United States adds to the stress.

Because the quality of foreign medical schools varies widely, it is important to consult graduates of the schools to which you apply. Write directly to each medical school and request the names of a few physician alumni in the United States with whom you could speak. If you ultimately choose to attend a foreign medical school, make every attempt to visit that school before matriculating. School catalogues may offer descriptions that make antiquated facilities sound state-of-the-art.

The goal of most students who enroll in foreign medical schools is to return to the United States either as transfer students to American medical schools or as physicians licensed to practice in this country. There are three common ways to do so.

Perhaps the most desirable route back home is by taking the Medical Sciences Knowledge Profile (MSKP), a test similar to Part I (the basic sciences portion) of the National Board Examination, the test which American students often take to obtain licensure to practice medicine. Students then forward the results of the examination to certain medical schools that may admit them as transfer students with advanced standing. During the academic year 1985-1986, of the thousands of Americans studying outside this country, only 289 successfully transferred to medical schools in the United States (Personal communication, AAMC staff member, March 1986).

Another way to return home is by completing a "Fifth Pathway." The Fifth Pathway allows some students who graduated from college in the United States and have not yet received their MD degrees to return to this country for one year of clinical training in a hospital program approved by the American Medical Association. Students who complete this year are given clearance to apply for internship and residency programs in the United States.

One of the benefits of the Fifth Pathway is that it allows accepted students to bypass some of the requirements for the MD peculiar to the nation in which they have studied. Medical students attending Universidad Autonoma de Guadalajara, for example, can avoid the year of social service which that school requires.

In 1985, of 554 foreign medical students with United States citizenship who applied for Fifth Pathway slots, 374 were accepted (Personal communication, AAMC staff member, March 1986).

Finally, students who have completed every requirement to practice medicine in the country in which they studied are eligible for certification by the Educational Commission for Foreign Medical Graduates (ECFMG). Certification allows these students to enter internships and residencies in the United States and is obtained by passing the Foreign Medical Graduate Examination in the Medical Sciences (FMGEMS). In July 1985, the basic sciences portion of the exam was taken by 2,910 American foreign medical graduates, and 20 percent passed. Of the 1,819 Americans who took the clinical sciences portion, 29 percent passed (Personal communication, ECFMG staff member, March 1986).

It is important to note that either a Fifth Pathway or satisfactory performance on the FMGEMS examination only provides the legal framework that allows a foreign medical graduate to serve an internship and residency in this country. He or she must still compete for these positions with graduates from American medical schools. In addition, all foreign medical graduates must also pass the Federation Licensing Examination (FLEX) before practicing medicine beyond the residency years.

The bottom line is that some Americans who study medicine in a foreign country never achieve the goal of becoming practicing physicians in the United States. Moreover, all indications are that it will get harder to reach that goal as pressure from American physicians to "close the door" on foreign medical graduates mounts. You must decide if your level of interest in the profession and your level of confidence are sufficient to sustain you through years of foreign study which can be extremely stressful and can end in disappointment. Knowing the risks, if you decide that becoming a physician is worth the price of pursuing your MD outside the United States, keep in mind that many competent American physicians have traveled the same road that you have chosen.

REFERENCES

1. As quoted in Allen RG: *Creating Wealth*. New York, Simon & Schuster, 1986, p 292.
2. Association of American Medical Colleges: Quality of preparation for the practice of medicine in certain foreign chartered medical schools. 56: 965-979, 1981.
3. World Health Organization: *World Directory of Medical Schools*. Geneva, World Health Organization, 1979.

10

Attending Medical School

"We are drowning in information but starved for knowledge" (1).

JOHN NAISBITT

THE EVOLUTION OF MEDICAL EDUCATION IN THE UNITED STATES

During the 19th century, medical schools in the United States were often no more than trade schools. For decades, most physicians were prepared for their profession by serving as apprentices to physicians already in practice. Although a few quality medical schools did exist (Pennsylvania, Columbia, Harvard, and Dartmouth), many were owned by small groups of physicians from Europe who often established their "proprietary" schools to make money. Some students in such schools had not completed high school.

But medical education began to change. The formation of the American Medical Association (1847) and the Association of American Medical Colleges (1876) provided an organized format in which educators could voice calls for improved standards. Both organizations strongly encouraged more rigorous physician training and licensing.

In 1889 and 1893, respectively, The Johns Hopkins Hospital and The Johns Hopkins School of Medicine were established. The new school required a college degree for admission and introduced a structured four-year program which included basic sciences (anatomy, physiology, etc.) and clinical experience as part of medical training. The curriculum, as well as the close ties between the hospital and medical school, reflected the German model of medical education which was well known to Johns Hopkins' first dean, Dr. William H. Welch. Many of the school's early graduates went on to other schools where they encouraged the adoption of the Hopkins approach.

Changing economics forced the closing of many medical schools in the early 1900s. State licensing boards started to require a longer period of training, discouraging some would-be physicians and reducing the number of student-customers. At the same time, new requirements that medical schools have modern laboratories and clinical facilities increased the overhead of operating a professional school beyond the means of proprietary institutions.

The next important advance was made in 1910 when Abraham Flexner of the Carnegie Foundation for the Advancement of Teaching published his report on the quality of education at each medical school in the United States. At the time of the report, entitled *Medical Education in the United States and Canada* (2), only 16 of the 155 medical schools required two years of college as an entrance requirement and most students had little contact with patients (3). Flexner recommended close ties between medical schools, universities, and hospitals. He viewed the Johns Hopkins system of medical education as a model and emphasized the need for previous training in biology, chemistry, and physics before entrance to medical school.

While many small medical colleges had already closed by 1910, Flexner's report hastened the decline of others. By 1915, the number of schools had fallen from 155 to 95 (4), and those still operating were moving toward the comprehensive model Flexner had proposed.

The focus of alarm shifted considerably in the following decades. The curricula of the surviving institutions became quite concentrated, especially with the mass of knowledge generated by scientific advances during the 1930s and 1940s. The dividends of physician research during World War II further increased the amount of material presented to medical students.

The increased information load and heightened emphasis on basic science, even at the level of premedical studies, never disappeared. Its intensity was, perhaps, diminished by the insistence of medical students during the 1960s that their education be tailored more toward the primary care needs of the community. But even today, ways to encourage more well-rounded premedical preparation and less potentially stifling medical education need to be explored.

In the 1980s, far from the situation in the early part of this century, the vast majority of medical students begin their professional training after receiving bachelor level degrees from accredited colleges. While different medical schools have different academic schedules, each divides its curriculum into classroom instruction in the basic sciences and clinical experience on hospital wards.

THE PRECLINICAL (BASIC SCIENCE) YEARS

The length of the basic science, or classroom, portion of your medical education will vary depending upon the school at which you study. Most medical schools divide their curricula in half, reserving the first two years mainly for classroom instruction before two years of clinical rotations in a hospital. Others, however, limit classroom training to seven quarters, and students begin clinical work during the spring of their second year. Duke University School of Medicine schedules the required basic sciences into just one year, but students most often return to the classroom for additional study later in their training.

The intent of basic science education is to provide you with the necessary knowledge for you to feel competent studying more advanced medical science and to allow you to understand and interpret clinical findings. Some schools organize this background material into body systems—the circulatory system, the respiratory system, the reproductive system, and others—and present the structure (anatomy, histology), function (physiology), and misfunction (pathophysiology, pathology) of each as a distinct unit. Other schools choose to use structure, function, and misfunction themselves as organizing principles. These institutions, for example, present the physiology of all body systems before moving on to pathophysiology.

Education in the basic sciences generally includes courses in anatomy, cell biology, embryology, genetics, histology, biochemistry, physiology, neurosciences, behavioral sciences, microbiology, pathology, pathophysiology, pharmacology, and clinical skills. Not every school's curriculum includes each of these, and many require others in subjects as diverse as medical jurisprudence, nutrition, medical ethics, and the history of medicine.

The topics covered by some courses are easy to guess from their names, but others are masked by course titles that may be unfamiliar to you. Each course is defined in the Glossary at the end of this book. Reading through the definitions will give you a better picture of the content of the basic sciences years in medical school.

Perhaps more important than understanding exactly what will be presented is understanding how the material will be presented. While problem-solving sessions and laboratories are also used, lectures are still the main way that instructors relate basic science to medical students. Professors typically speak for one hour, almost always using slides rather than blackboards, to convey theories or data.

Attending lecture after lecture can make the day seem very long. My friends and I often despaired at the lack of creativity demonstrated by a curriculum that sometimes scheduled six lectures in a row. Listening passively to physicians giving their talks in an auditorium, we felt, made much of the material presented seem dull. Moreover, once we began our clinical rotations, we saw more clearly the very real applicability of the basic sciences to the practice of medicine and regretted that they were presented in a fashion that limited their practical application.

Like it or not, however, medical schools change slowly. Innovative teaching methods and curricula that encourage more independent study by students have not yet come into widespread use in the training of American physicians. Similar to my friends and me, you may find yourself looking anxiously past the basic science years and toward clinical work.

THE CLINICAL YEARS

The clinical years of medical school are made up of rotations spent working on hospital wards and in clinics. Each rotation generally lasts between four and nine weeks and concentrates on one medical specialty. Completion of several specific rotations is required for graduation, but time is also available for elective rotations in areas of special interest to you.

The required clerkships generally include internal medicine, surgery, pediatrics, obstetrics/gynecology, and psychiatry. Some schools require other rotations in areas such as neurology, ophthalmology, and family medicine. Since these and other medical specialty names may be unfamiliar to you, they are included in the Glossary at the end of this book.

While lectures are often given during clerkships, the focus of each is patient care. Students interview patients in order to write the histories of their illnesses and continue to monitor the patients' progress while in the hospital. Students also draw blood, learn to analyze urine, and may assist with, or actually perform, other procedures such as sampling the fluid that surrounds the spinal cord (a procedure known as a lumbar puncture, or "LP").

For at least some of the clerkships, students "take call," staying overnight in the hospital to help interns and residents with patient care. The internal medicine (or "medicine") clerkship and the surgery clerkship are noted for their particularly demanding schedules. At many schools, students take call every third night during these two rotations and may remain until fairly late in the evening even when not "on call." Other required clerkships, such as psychiatry, generally require less of a time commitment.

What each clerkship shares in common, and the reason why students often find the clinical years much more enjoyable than the basic science years, is student participation in the care of patients. Textbooks change from study aids for next week's biochemistry exam to resources used to review the facts known about an illness besieging today's patient. Knowledge of anatomy changes from a way to perform a cadaver's dissection to a way of understanding why drawing arterial blood from the wrong site can severely injure your patient.

Another agenda for the clinical years is your selection of a particular field of interest. By the end of your third year of medical school, you will need to decide what kind of physician you wish to become. Shortly thereafter, you will need to apply for a residency (further training in a specific area of the medical profession). Residencies are available in each medical specialty. Every practicing surgeon has completed a surgical residency and each practicing psychiatrist has completed a psychiatry residency.

Students explore different fields in medicine by doing elective rotations. A student with an interest in becoming a surgeon, for example, might spend several extra months (beyond those included in the required surgery rotation) working on the surgical wards. Someone with an interest in pediatrics might spend a month working at a city clinic where infants and children are treated. Elective time may also be spent doing medical research.

Whatever specific academic program you structure, working with patients within the doctor-patient relationship will allow you to understand their concerns and will make you privy to the most intimate details of their lives. If you take the time to listen, people from backgrounds wholly different from your own will often reveal more and more of themselves. Interacting with individuals and their families during difficult times will make you a part of the drama of human existence and will provide you with the opportunity to make a real difference in their lives.

EMOTIONAL SUPPORT SYSTEMS

Beginning medical school can be both exciting and traumatic: exciting because all of the effort in premedical courses, all of the preparation for the MCAT, and all of the anxiety waiting for letters of acceptance have paid off, and a career in medicine is nearly assured; traumatic because the start of professional training means new classmates, often a new city, and certainly a more focused and time-intensive academic schedule.

I and many students with whom I have spoken adjusted to our new colleagues and our new homes quickly. But it took longer to come to terms with medical education itself. The large volume of information presented during the first two years of medical school demanded rote memorization rather than independent thinking. The heavy workload, which seemed to devour any hope of free time, made many of us feel that the interpersonal skills and outside interests we most valued would be lost. Contact with patients was nearly nonexistent until the last quarter of the second year, and some students began to doubt that medicine really was the human profession for which they had hoped.

What made things worse was that few of us knew at the time that our feelings of anxiety and even depression were shared by many others in the class. Young people in a new social setting often find it difficult to communicate their fears, and it wasn't until the second year that we shared openly with each other how difficult and stressful the first year of medical school had been.

The fact is that feelings of anxiety, fear, and low mood are most often a reflection of the shortcomings of medical education rather than the shortcomings of students. Such feelings are an understandable response to a threatening environment.

The very real pressures of medical education make what I like to call support systems extremely important. Support systems are really just networks of people with whom you can talk openly about your problems and in whom you feel comfortable placing your trust. For me, my parents fulfilled the role. They listened attentively to all my concerns and fears during hours of phone calls home. Close friends also understood the extent to which the first year of medical school was affecting me. Even more valuable than the advice they offered was the opportunity they provided me to vent my feelings.

Caring people are more available than you might think. Parents and friends from home are obvious sources of support, but a professor who has earned your respect or a dean dealing with student concerns is also a valuable resource. New-found friends in medical school will often be willing to listen. They may be wrestling, as my classmates were, with the same feelings you need to talk about. Sharing your thoughts can help everyone involved.

Even with support systems, one can lose perspective and feel locked into a painful environment. Seemingly insurmountable challenges and the fear of failure weigh heavily on students used to high achievement. Professional psychiatric counseling is usually available to medical students and can take the edge off during particularly difficult times. Don't go it alone.

PRESERVING OUTSIDE INTERESTS

As I discussed above, perhaps the most stressful element of my first year of medical school was the fear that I was becoming unidimensional—leaving my special nonmedical interests and skills behind forever. One of the keys to maintaining perspective is understanding that the activities you truly value, while they might need to be curtailed for a year or two, need not remain in storage forever. By staying close enough in touch with outside interests, much of the panic created by intense professional training can be avoided.

Just as putting aside free time is helpful to combat the college "premed syndrome," allotting a number of hours each week as time reserved for nonmedical interests can make medical school more tolerable. This reserved time may translate to reading a novel for an hour each evening or to going out dancing every Friday night. It may mean signing on with an intramural volleyball team or signing up for ballroom dance classes. However the time is used, it will provide a release from memorizing biochemical pathways and anatomical landmarks. Remember, clearing your mind now and then will make it easier to achieve academically.

It is also helpful to make certain that the nonmedical skills you value will be used in the near future and not become stale. Scheduling summer employment which will call these skills into play can set your mind at ease. If you fear that your knowledge of art history is slipping away, apply for a job at a museum or an art gallery. Demonstrating your resolve to remain a well-rounded person is a reassuring signal to yourself that the intensity of medical education cannot rob you of your diversity.

Physicians who have continued to pursue outside interests similar to your own are another potential source of reassurance. Doctors are involved in government, journalism, music, and many other areas. While you may or may not come into personal contact with these multidimensional professionals as you move through medical school, you should feel free to write to physicians well-known for their achievements outside the field. They will generally be eager to offer advice and encouragement.

Finally, as you fight to stay whole, resolve not to forget how difficult the struggle can sometimes be. In the future, if enough of us who become professors and deans remember our feelings as first- and second-year medical students, perhaps we will change medical education for the better.

REFERENCES

1. Naisbitt J: *Megatrends.* New York, Warner Books, 1984.
2. Flexner A: *Medical Education in the United States and Canada.* Boston, The Merrymount Press, 1910.
3. American Medical Association: *Future Directions for Medical Education.* Chicago, American Medical Association, 1982, pp 59-60.
4. Starr P: *The Social Transformation of American Medicine.* New York, Basic Books, 1982, p 120.

Conclusions

"People are just as loving and kind and honest as they ever were and helping them is still worth it. It's worth every bit of it."

DR. KARL MECH, SR.*

Many times, while writing this book, I reflected on my high school, college, and medical school years. I imagined myself reading these pages and made sure that they addressed the many questions and the many doubts I had at each stage of my preparation for a career in medicine.

By my doing so, *Medical School: Getting In, Staying In, Staying Human* has become not only a complete guide to the medical school admissions process, but also a guide through the highs and lows of premedical and medical education.

As you encounter those highs and lows, I would be interested in hearing about your experiences. Feel free to write to me at P.O. Box 541, Marblehead, MA 01945.

---

*Dr. Karl Mech, Sr. is a past president of the Maryland Medical Association. He shared with me his thoughts on the future of medical practice during a personal interview (March 1986).

Glossary

AAMC See Association of American Medical Colleges.

Aerospace Medicine A medical specialty. Practitioners of aerospace medicine address the health needs of those intimately involved with air and space travel.

AMA See American Medical Association.

AMCAS See American Medical College Application Service.

American Medical Association (AMA) A professional association representing many thousands of physicians in the United States.

American Medical College Application Service (AMCAS) A branch of the American Association of Medical Colleges (AAMC) that publishes a standard application form. Medical school applicants may fill out the AMCAS application, and AMCAS will forward it (for a fee) to any participating medical school the applicant designates.

Anatomy The science or study of the structure of the animal body. A course in human anatomy is a required part of the first year medical school curriculum. Students most often spend long laboratory hours dissecting dead bodies, called cadavers.

Anesthesiology A medical specialty. Anesthesiologists are skilled in the use of drugs that alter a patient's state of consciousness and ability to feel pain so that surgical procedures can be performed.

Association of American Medical Colleges (AAMC) The organization that represents medical schools in the United

States and Canada and formulates guidelines for the medical school admissions process. Undertakes frequent studies of premedical and medical education. Publishers of *Medical School Admission Requirements.*

BA-MD Program   A combined college/medical school program that students begin after high school. BA-MD programs generally last six or seven years. Accepted students enjoy the security of conditional admission to medical school even before they begin undergraduate study.

Biochemistry   The study of the chemical substances and reactions in the body which allow normal function and contribute to disease. A course in biochemistry is a required part of the first year medical school curriculum.

Cadaver   A dead body. Medical students generally dissect cadavers as part of their required medical school course in human anatomy.

Cardiology   A medical specialty. Cardiologists treat diseases of the heart.

Child Psychiatry   A medical specialty. Child psychiatrists treat mental illness in children.

Colon and Rectal Surgery   A medical specialty. Colon and rectal surgeons perform operations to treat disease or injury in the lowest part of the digestive tract.

Dermatology   A medical specialty. Dermatologists treat diseases of the skin.

ECFMG   See Educational Commission for Foreign Medical Graduates.

Educational Commission for Foreign Medical Graduates (ECFMG)   An organization that provides information to graduates of foreign medical schools and administers the Foreign Medical Graduate Examination in the Medical Sciences (FMGEMS).

Elective   A rotation or other learning experience that a medical student schedules during his or her clinical years. No particular elective is required, but students must complete a certain number for credit toward graduation. A student interested in neurosurgery, for example, might schedule elective time to complete research in that area or to work an additional month with neurosurgeons.

Embryology   The study of the body's earliest development before birth. A course in embryology is a required part of the first year curriculum of many medical schools.

Emergency Medicine   A medical specialty. Emergency medicine physicians provide emergency medical care. A course covering the basic principles of emergency medicine is a required part of the first year curriculum of some medical schools.

Endocrinology   A medical specialty. Endocrinologists treat disorders of glands and their secretions.

Epidemiology   The study of the factors influencing the spread of disease. A course in epidemiology is a required part of the second year curriculum of some medical schools.

Family Practice   A medical specialty. Family practitioners attend to the general health needs of all family members. Family practice residencies include training in family dynamics and family planning.

Federation Licensing Examination (FLEX)   The FLEX examination, developed by the Federation of State Medical Boards, is used by all 50 states to license physicians to practice medicine.

Fifth Pathway   A year of clinical training at an American medical school for which Americans studying medicine outside the United States may apply. Students who complete a Fifth Pathway are given clearance to apply for internship and residency positions in the United States.

FLEX   See Federation Licensing Examination.

FMG   See Foreign Medical Graduate.

FMGEMS   See Foreign Medical Graduate Examination in the Medical Sciences.

Foreign Medical Graduate (FMG)   A graduate of a medical school outside the United States. The term refers not only to foreigners who graduate from foreign medical schools, but also to Americans who complete their studies outside this country.

Foreign Medical Graduate Examination in the Medical Sciences (FMGEMS)   The examination administered by the Educational Commission for Foreign Medical Graduates (ECFMG) that foreign medical graduates (FMGs) must pass to obtain ECFMG certification. Certification allows FMGs to enter internships and residencies in the United States.

Gastroenterology   A medical specialty. Gastroenterologists specialize in the treatment of diseases of the digestive tract, including the stomach and intestines.

Genetics   The study of the mechanisms by which traits are passed from generation to generation. A course in genetics is a required part of either the first or second year curriculum of some medical schools.

GPA   See Grade Point Average.

Grade Point Average (GPA)   A numerical representation of the average of a student's grades.

Gynecology   A medical specialty. Gynecologists treat diseases of the female reproductive tract, including the vagina, ovaries, and uterus. A clinical rotation in gynecology is a required part of the medical school curriculum.

Hematology   A medical specialty. Hematologists treat disorders of the blood.

Histology   The science or study of the microscopic structure of body tissues. A course in histology is a required part of the first year medical school curriculum.

Immunology   A medical specialty. Immunologists treat illnesses in which the immune system, the body's surveillance system against infection (among other things), is centrally involved. A course in immunology is a required part of either the first or second year curriculum of some medical schools.

Infectious Disease   A medical specialty. Physicians specializing in infectious disease treat illnesses caused by organisms that invade the human body. These organisms range from tiny viruses to relatively large parasitic worms.

Intern   A physician completing the first year of training after medical school. Interns are responsible for the care of patients in the hospital and are paid for their services.

Internal Medicine   A medical specialty. Doctors of internal medicine (internists) treat the broad range of illnesses that affect the internal organs of the body.

Internship   An outdated term which is still frequently used to refer to the first year of postgraduate training for physicians.

MCAT   See Medical College Admission Test.

MD-PhD   Doctor of Medicine-Doctor of Philosophy. A term generally used to refer to an individual who has earned advanced degrees in both medicine and a basic science, such as biochemistry or genetics.

Medical College Admission Test   A 6½-hour exam covering biology, chemistry, and physics. Taking the MCAT is a requirement for admission to most medical schools in the United States, and an applicant's scores can greatly influence his or her chances of acceptance.

Medical Ethics   The study of the moral issues, such as those surrounding euthanasia, that are involved in medical care and medical research. A course in medical ethics is a required part of the curriculum of a small number of medical schools.

Medical Sciences Knowledge Profile (MSKP)   An examination covering basic sciences which is similar to Part I of the National Board Examination. This exam is taken by many medical students studying outside the United States in the hope that a strong performance on the exam will improve their chances of transferring to American medical schools.

Medical Scientist Training Program (MSTP)   A program supported by the National Institute of General Medical Sciences which offers exceptional students financial support while they pursue combined MD-PhD degrees.

Microbiology   The science and study of microorganisms, such as viruses and bacteria. A course in microbiology is part of the required first or second year curriculum of many medical schools.

MSKP   See Medical Sciences Knowledge Profile.

MSTP   See Medical Scientist Training Program.

National Board Examination   One of the tests that American medical students may take to obtain licensure to practice medicine.

Neonatology   A medical specialty. Neonatologists treat illnesses in newborn infants.

Nephrology   A medical specialty. Nephrologists treat illnesses affecting the kidneys.

Neurology   A medical specialty. Neurologists treat illnesses affecting the nervous system.

Neurosurgery   A medical specialty. Neurosurgeons operate on damaged or diseased structures in the nervous system.

Nuclear Medicine   A medical specialty. Physicians who practice nuclear medicine use radioactive particles to diagnose and treat illness.

Obstetrics   A medical specialty. Obstetricians take care of pregnant women and deliver babies.

Oncology   A medical specialty. Oncologists treat patients who have tumors.

Ophthalmology   A medical specialty. Ophthalmologists treat illnesses affecting the eyes.

Orthopedic Surgery   A medical specialty. Orthopedic surgeons specialize in the treatment of bone and joint abnormalities.

Otolaryngology   A medical specialty. Otolaryngologists specialize in the medical and surgical treatment of disease in the ears, nose, and throat.

Pathology   A medical specialty. Pathologists identify abnormalities in tissue specimens taken from patients with suspected disease and from cadavers at autopsy. A course in pathology is a required part of the medical school curriculum.

Pathophysiology The science and study of how bodily functions become disordered and contribute to disease. All medical school curricula include teaching on pathophysiology, but not always as a separate course.

Pediatrics A medical specialty. Pediatricians care for infants and children.

Pharmacology The science or study of the interactions of drugs with the body. A course in pharmacology is a required part of the second year curriculum of most medical schools.

Plastic Surgery A medical specialty. Plastic surgeons repair or reshape body structures.

Premedical Syndrome A mindset that besieges some premedical students, including an apparent lack of interest in activities outside the requirements of the premedical curriculum. Premedical syndrome reflects the demands and uncertainties of premedical education, not any inherent weakness in those afflicted.

Psychiatry A medical specialty. Psychiatrists treat patients suffering from mental illness.

Public Health The discipline that addresses the health of the community as a whole.

Radiology A medical specialty. Radiologists diagnose illness using imaging techniques that allow them to visualize structures inside the body. Some radiologists actually treat diseases, such as cancer, using precise amounts of radiation to kill of abnormal cells.

Residency The hospital-based program that trains a physician in a particular field of medicine by allowing him or her increasing responsibility for patient care.

Resident A physician serving a residency. Residents are responsible for the care of patients in the hospital and are paid for their services.

Rotation A period of weeks or months during the clinical years of medical school when students learn about a particular field of medicine by working with physicians who practice that type of medicine.

Surgery   A medical specialty. Surgeons perform operations in the treatment of injury and illness.

Urology   A medical specialty. Urologists treat illnesses that involve the urinary tract in both men and women and the genital area in men.

Appendix

Medical Schools Offering a Combined BA-MD Program to Graduating High School Seniors, 1984-85*

In collaboration with the university's own undergraduate school:

Boston University School of Medicine

Brown University Program in Medicine

Case Western Reserve University School of Medicine

Howard University College of Medicine

Louisiana State University School of Medicine in Shreveport †

---

*Data from *Medical School Admissions Requirements, 1986-87,* published by the Association of American Medical Colleges.

†Program admits only state residents.

University of Miami School of Medicine
University of Michigan Medical School
University of Missouri–Kansas City School of Medicine
Northwestern University Medical School
Northeastern Ohio Universities College of Medicine †

In collaboration with other undergraduate schools:

Albany Medical College of Union University
University of California, Los Angeles
Hahnemann University School of Medicine †
Jefferson Medical College of Thomas Jefferson University
SUNY Downstate Medical Center College of Medicine †
Medical College of Pennsylvania
Ponce School of Medicine
Medical College of Wisconsin